HOW to Become a HOLY Man!

(40 Good Reasons WHY People Should FAST and PRAY!)

By
The Worldwide People's Revolution!®

Book 045

(A Painting of a Holy Man from the 1400's)

Copyright Dedication and Introduction

By
Dr. Samuel Walker Edison, Ph.D., MA, BS, and QC!

ISBN — 13: 978-1541-3928-47

ISBN — 10: 1541-3928-41

00-02 [_] This Inspired Book is now DEDICATED to **"The Swanky Association of Truth Seekers and Treasure Hunters, Worldwide!"** We Trust that you are one of them. May the Power of God be with you.

00-03 [_] Fasting and Praying is not a very Popular Thing in **"The Divided States of United Lies,"** nor even in most Western "Civilized" Societies, who Judge themselves to be Superior to Adam, Abraham, Melchizedek, Isaac, Jacob, Joseph, Moses, Elijah, King David, Isaiah, Jeremiah, Ezekiel, Daniel, Joel, Amos, Jesus, John, Peter, Paul, James, and all of the other Saints who did much Fasting and Praying, which was the ONE THING that all Saints did, in spite of whatever else that they might have done, which is also True for our Elected King, who has done much Fasting and Praying. In Fact, the most Fasting that he did at any one given Time, was 314 Days in only 14 Months, after which he was "as Strong as Samson," you might say: beCause he could Lift very Heavy Rocks with the Greatest of Ease, as if they were no Heavier than common Red Bricks! Moreover, to Back Up such Claims, he and his Brother Vern Built some Amazing Stone Houses with Large Rough Rocks, which you can See Photographs of on the Covers of Future Books that **The Worldwide People's Revolution!®** shall surely Publish for your Enlightenment, Education and Entertainment — that is, IF the "Military Industrial Congressional News Media Red Jew Bankers' COMPLEX" does not get in the Way of it! After all, Provable Truths are a Great Threat to the Evil Empire, which is Controlled by those Lying Red Jews, who were also the Enemies of Jesus Christ and his Self-disciplined Disciples, whom Jesus referred to as *"the Synagogue of Satan,"* in *Revelation 2:9 and 3:9:* beCause they call themselves Jews; but, they do not have the Spirit of Father Abraham. Indeed, they do the Works of their Evil Stepfather, the Devil, himself.

00-04 [_] For Example, our Elected King's old Computer quit working: beCause of a Bad Switch for getting it Started, which the Apple Store wanted to Repair for only $999.98, even though the entire Computer was only $3,599.98 to begin with, and the Switch might have Cost all of 2$. However, even if it Costed 20$, and required all of 2 Hours to Replace it: beCause of the Built-in Complications of Capitalism, that would amount to a Total of only 60$, even at the Rate of 20$ per Hour for their "Services," in spite of the Fact that the Service Repair Man revealed that he was only getting $16.15 per Hour, which barely made it Possible for him to Live! Therefore, one might Rightly Ask, "WHO was getting the Extra 800+ Dollars for Repairing such Switches?"

00-05 [_] Well, of course, you could say that all such Money was to Cover the Costs of "Overhead," as in the Capitalist Banners that were Flying over the Heads of the American Bisons for thousands of Years before Europeans arrived, which no Bisons could Live without. For Example, those Bisons had to have ElecTrickery in their Houses, even if they did not have Computers of any Kinds. Nevertheless, our Elected King was Naturally Stranded with a "Broke-down" Computer, and was Perplexed for what to Do about it: beCause of Spending his Money on other Necessities for Living — such as a Roof over his Head and Bed. Therefore, he Attempted to Write this Document on another Mac Computer, and Save it to a little Computer Chip, which Rejected the Idea: beCause the Computer was Old, and could not Discover any Way to make it "Compatible" with a Modern Computer Chip without Connecting to the Internet, which he did not Want to Do: beCause a Connection with the Internet would Defile the Computer beyond Repair, whereby it would become Worthless for anyone to Watch Old DVD's on it: beCause of getting "Updated" by Satan and Sons, Incorporated, who know HOW to make those Old DVD's Obsolete, in spite of being only 10 Years or so Old, which Costed several thousands of Dollars for Nature Programs and Old Movies, etc., etc.

00-06 [_] So, O Doctor Edison, could the Document not be Downloaded from one Computer Directly into the other Computer, after it got Repaired for $999.98? Moreover, why did they not just Charge an even 1,000$ for the Repairs of the 2$ Switch?

00-07 [_] Well, the Objective was to Force our Elected King, and almost everyone else, to Buy what they call a "Service Agreement," which is Designed to Cover all Future Repairs on such Machines. For Example, they Wanted $299.98 per Year for the "Service Agreement" for the Old Mac Computer, times 10 Years, equals no less than $2,999.80! — except that those "Service Agreement" Costs would naturally go UP each Year, whereby the Buyer might have to Pay for the Machine 2 or 3 Times, just by Buying into that Capitalist SCAM. After all, the entire Computer might have Actually Costed as little as 550$: beCause of Mass-producing them by Cheap Labor in China, where those Work Slaves might get as little as 2$ per Hour for their Services! Moreover, they dare not Complain about their Wages: beCause there are a Billion Unemployed Slaves patiently waiting to get their Jobs in Vietnam, Cambodia, Laos, Burma, Ecuador, Guatemala, Honduras, Nicaragua, El Salvador, Mexico, Ireland, Iceland, Greenland, or wherever around the World: beCause that is **"The Nature of CAPITALISM!" (A List of the EVILS of CAPITALISM!) By The Worldwide People's Revolution!®**

00-08 [_] So, O Doctor Edison, it seems as though this is a "No Win" Capitalist Game that we are now Playing, whereby almost no one is Free to Do any Fasting nor even Praying in Peace: beCause of those Endless BILLS to be Paid! Indeed, WHEN and WHERE would a Normal Person Do any Fasting: seeing that there are Debts to be Paid? Therefore, HOW is anyone going to become a HOLY Man?

00-09 [_] Well, that is a very Good Question, which does have a Good Answer; but, only IF **The Worldwide People's Revolution!®** can get **"The New RIGHTEOUS One-World Government"** Established, which will Assist almost everyone to Accomplish it, with the Exceptions of People who do not Want to Do any Fasting, or who Live in such Remote Places on the Earth, that no one in the Civilized World can Contact them, which is Okay: beCause only a very Small Percentage of the Masses of People are Sincerely Interested in Doing any Fasting. After all, X-amount of People are already Healthy and Happy, they say, who have little or no Interest in it — that is, until they get Deathly Sick or Badly Wounded; and then they have no other Options, except to Do like the American Bisons used to Do, if they got Wounded or Sick. Indeed, there was and still is a Natural Remedy for all Ailments, which was Workable for all Creatures Great and Small, which was to STOP EATING whenever they Lost their Appetites.

00-10 [_] O Doctor Sam, would it not be Wiser to Visit a Medical Doctor, who might be Able to Prescribe some Magic Pill, Potion, or Lotion, which might Cure any Ailments — and for less than the Repair Bill on that Computer, plus or minus (±) a few hundred thousand almost worthless American dollars? For Example, I have a middle-aged Friend, who Ate like a Hog for 40+ Years, and finally got his Heart Attack, which Automatically put him into the Loving Hands of Lying Red Jew Medical Doctors, who Charged him upwards of a Million Dollars: beCause he did not have ObamaScare Medical Insurance: beCause he could not Afford "Health Care." And I Ask him, "How in the World did you Think that you could get by with Committing such Horrible Dietary SINS for 40+ Years, without Reaping what you Sowed, as the Apostle Paul put it? Yes, he wrote, *'Be not Deceived by any Means: beCause, as a Man Sows, so shall he Reap; and therefore, he or she who Sows Seeds of Lusts and Greed, shall Reap Sicknesses, Diseases, Accidents, Divorces, Heartaches, Sorrows, and all Kinds of Ailments.' — The New MAGNIFIED Version in Plain English.*" And he said, "I never Thought of it. Moreover, none of the Public School Teachers, nor even the Sunday School Teachers, ever Mentioned a Thing about Dietary Sins. In Fact, not even the Irreverent Jelly Belly from the Unholy Church of Dietary Sinners ever Mentioned it: beCause they are Chief Friends of the Church of Picnics, who Love to EAT — nay, to FEAST on the Dead Carcasses of BEASTS: beCause it is their TRADITION to do so; and God Forbid that any of them should Question their Vain Traditions of Men, including any Eating Habits. However, to make Matters Worse by a hundred Times, Modern Capitalists have ADDED tens of thousands of Chemical Abominations to our Foods and Drinks, in order to Enhance the Flavors, and to get Weak-minded People Addicted to all such Foods and Drinks."

00-11 [_] And I said, "Sir, it must be Time to Take Back America from the Military Industrial Congressional News Media Bankers' Complex Economic System of Suicide, and Establish **'The New RIGHTEOUS One-World Government!' (HOW to Establish a Righteous One-World Government without Going to WAR!) By The Worldwide People's Revolution!®**" And he said, "I have no Idea what you Mean by the Military Industrial Congressional News Media Bankers' Complex, let alone an Economic System of Self-promoted Suicide: beCause I have not

Studied: **'The Great False Economy is now DEBUNKED!' (Adolf Hitler had a much Better Economic System!) By The Worldwide People's Revolution!**® Indeed, that would Require Time and Patience, which I do not have: beCause I have BILLS to be Paid. Moreover, if I did not get those Bills Paid, my Wife would just Naturally DIVORCE me; and then what would I do for SEX, which is the Chief Reason for Living!?"

00-12 [_] And I said, "There is much more to Life than having Sex. In Fact, according to the *Holy Bible,* Jesus Christ Lived for 34 Years and 4 Days without having any Sex, if you can Believe it." And he said, "I do not Believe it. First of all, he would have Suffered with Swollen Testicles, which are sometimes called 'blue balls,' which, if not Treated by having Ejaculations, will Result with Testicular Cancer: beCause it is Unnatural for a Man to not have Sex in one Form or another, which is also True of all Mammals: beCause it is the Way that we were Designed by some Great Master Mind, whom we may call 'God,' which Means 'Supreme Ruler,' or 'Divine Lawmaker,' who Created Natural LAWS, without which there would be NO World to Live in, much less such a Well-Organized World as this, whereby Nature Works in Perfect Harmony with Natural Laws and Flexible Rules."

00-13 [_] And I said, "Would that Great Creator God be the same one who Proclaimed himself to be the God of Abraham, Isaac, and Jacob?" And he said, "Well, Jehovah God does seem to be quite Unaware of most Natural Laws. For Example, in his World, the Earth is at the Center of the Universe, and the Stars were Created as an Afterthought, even as the Sunstar was Created after the Earth was Created, according to *Genesis 1,* which is a bit Confusing, if not Totally Perplexing and Bewildering: beCause, in the Real World, this Earth is Located in a Minor Solar System, with just an Ordinary Sunstar, which would Certainly NOT Qualify this Solar System to have Divine Powers over ALL other Solar Systems, Nebulas, Galaxies, and so on. In Fact, it would be Fair to say that Disregarding the Unholy Mutilated Bible, this Solar System is of no Great Significance at all, even within this Galaxy, which is also a Minor Galaxy, when Compared with Major Galaxies, which might be a thousand Times as BIG as this Galaxy. Therefore, it is Irrational to Think that this Tiny Earth might be the Eternal Home of the Great Creator God, who has Legions of Holy Angels at his Command, who would more likely Live within Jupiter, than within the Hollow Earth: beCause Jupiter is like a thousand Times as BIG!"

00-14 [_] And I said, "Does any of that Information have any Connection with WHY People should FAST and PRAY?" And he Answered, "Well, if we are Seeking Positions within the Holy Kingdom of All that is GOOD, I would say that that Information has Direct Connections with the Subjects within this Inspired Book." {See www.Amazon.com for: **"The Secret City of the Great King!" (HOW the True Church will Escape from the Great Tribulation!) By The Worldwide People's Revolution!**®

The Menu for a Feast of Fascinating Subjects

— Chapter 01 —

Understanding the Human Body

01-01 [_] O Elected King, I Wish to God that there were some Chapters telling about HOW to Understand the Human MIND, since the Human Body is quite easy to Understand, if you Study it; but, the Mind is an Impossible Thing for anyone to Understand — such as that Nonsense about the Earth being HOLLOW, and the Moon being Born from the Earth several Billion Years Ago, which left it Hollow, which you Claim to be the Headquarter of **"The New RIGHTEOUS One-World Government,"** seeing that Jesus Christ is the Great King, himself, who is Referred to in *Psalms 48, 50, and 87,* which are telling about *Mount Zion,* which is the Holy City of the Great King, which you Falsely Claim has been there, all along, which has yet to be Discovered by the Masses of People in this World of Woes, even though you say that it has been Discovered and Covered Up by several Governments of this World: beCause they do not Want the Masses of People to Learn that there are Far Advanced Civilizations within the Hollow Earth, which is where most of the UFO's (Unidentified Flying Objects) come from. Indeed, there have been tens of thousands of Sightings of all such UFO's, which the Anti-Christ False Cover-up Federal Government of **"The Divided States of United Lies"** has been Denying for a hundred or more Years: beCAUSE they Fear that they might be put Out of Business, if the Masses of People should Learn about *Mount Zion,* which has ZERO Taxes, ZERO Pollution, ZERO Criminals, ZERO Prisons, ZERO Election Deceptions, ZERO Drugs, ZERO Diseases, and so on. After all, the Biggest Businesses in America are Related with DRUGS, and Addictions of Various Kinds, including the Addictions that People have for Driving Cars, Pickups, Vans, Trucks, Buses, Motorcycles, Motor Scooters, Snowmobiles, and AIRPLANES, which are Abominations in the Nostrils of God and his Holy Angels, which should also be Abominations to all of us: beCause they are Contaminating the whole Earth, and so much so as to RUIN our Natural Environment! †§‡

01-02 [_] Well, my Friend, if you have "red" my other Inspired Books, you have Surely Learned about: **"The Great Worldwide TELEVISED Court HEARING!" (That Great Meeting of the Most Intelligent Minds!) By The Worldwide People's Revolution!®** Book 041. Indeed, if there is such a Beautiful City, Inside of a Hollow Earth, we will Discover it, even if We, The People, must Open Up all of the "Top Secret" Files of the Wicked Anti-Christ FALSE Cover-up Federal Governments of the World! Yes, *"There is nothing Secret that shall not be Revealed,"* as Jesus Explained: beCause it is our Judgment Day, and the Great KING of Kings will be in Charge of it! Therefore, have Faith in it.

01-03 [_] O Elected King, I do not have any Faith in anything that People Say nor Do: beCause they are not Perfectly Honest about anything.

01-04 [_] Well, I am now going to be Perfectly Honest with everyone about the Human Body, which Medical Science is Welcome to Prove to be True or False. Moreover, I Challenge anyone on this Earth to Prove my Inspired Words of Provable Truths to be WRong about any Subject;

and, if those Words are Proven to be WRong, we will simply Change them, and thus make them Correct, which is what Computers are Good for. After all, not even the *Holy Bible* is Accurate concerning several Important Subjects, which Need to be Corrected, which is WHY there are more than 200 English Versions of it: beCause People have been Attempting to Correct it. However, there is no Way to Correct a RED JEW LIE, except to simply Confess that it IS a Lie. For Example, I have already Proven by Means of Reason and Logic within other Inspired Books that the Noah's Ark Story is Basically a Jewish Fairy Tale, which will Prove to be most Interesting at **"The Great Worldwide TELEVISED Court HEARING!"**

01-05 [ ] O Elected King, suppose you and **The Worldwide People's Revolution!®** manage to DEBUNK the entire *Bible,* even as you have already Debunked *The Book of Mormon,* which is another Jewish Fairy Tale, what will you Replace that *Holy Bible* with, seeing that People Need some God to Look Up to?

01-06 [ ] Well, they will always have some Great Creator God to Look Up to, no matter how many Fairy Tales have been Debunked: beCause it is Impossible to have a Law without a Lawmaker, as I have stated before. Indeed, we cannot even have Traffic Laws without Lawmakers. Therefore, how much more must we Respect and Honor the Great Creator God, who Designed and Created EYEBALLS, for Example, which are very Complicated Things, we must Confess, which are Interconnected with many other very Complicated Parts of the Body, which Scientists have hardly Begun to Explore: beCause each Part is a little Universe of its own, which cannot even be Explained without THEORIES. For Example, just one Evil Thought can Effect the entire Body in a Bad Way, even as just one Good Thought can also Effect it in a Good Way. Yes, just some Good News in your Ears can make you Happy, while some Bad News can make you Unhappy. For Example, if you Received a Million-dollar Check in the Mail, and it Cashed at the Bank, you might be Elated by it, and so much so as to Forget all of your Troubles for at least one Day, whereby Wishful Dreams might be made Possible, which would Build Up your HOPES for a Better World — at least for YOUR World, which is a World within a World.

01-07 [ ] The Human Body is Basically a PIPE System, having thousands of Miles of little Pipes, called Blood Vessels, which Distribute Nourishment to all Parts of the Body, which Nourishment comes for the Air we Breathe, the Water we Drink, and the Foods that we Eat — all of which can be Greatly Effected by our THOUGHTS: beCause, *"As a Man Thinks, so is he,"* even as King Solomon Warned. Therefore, we must be Careful HOW we Think, and WHAT we Think about: beCause our Thoughts can Give to us Life or Death, which come in Degrees, beginning with Sicknesses and Diseases, which also come in Degrees — IN AS MUCH AS we Think and Act According to certain NATURAL and SPIRITUAL LAWS. Indeed, the Natural Laws are somewhat Visible, while the Spiritual Laws are somewhat Invisible; but, both are for Real, even if People Deny their Existence, even as the Earth is HOLLOW: beCause the Tree of Life did not DIE, nor was the Garden of Eden Destroyed by any Means; but, the Angels with the Flaming Swords still Guard it, whereby only HOLY People can Discover it, who are those Wise People, who have Humbled themselves by Means of Fasting and Praying, until they have become like Innocent Children with Pure Minds and Clean Bodies, which is no Easy Thing to Do, or else we would all be SAINTS, who could Walk on the Water with Jesus Christ.

01-08 [_] O Elected King, I find it Interesting that the Plumbing Systems of the Human Body, as well as that of all Mammals, was Designed for certain Kinds of Diets. For Example, you would never See a Horse Chasing after a Rabbit for Supper: beCause no Horse has an Appetite for Eating Rabbits, even as no Rabbit has an Appetite for Eating Snakes, Mice, Beatles, nor Bugs of any Kind, while Opossums, Raccoons, Skunks, and many other Creatures might Eat almost anything that Creeps, Runs, Flies, Digs, or Crawls: beCause that is HOW they were Designed. Therefore, since People can and do Eat just about everything on the Earth, including Glass and Nails, is it Fair to say that God Created us just a little Lower than Opossums, Raccoons, Skunks, and Snakes? After all, a Royal Heavenly Diet for Holy Angels would Surely be nothing less than Manna, or the Sweet Fruits from the Tree of Life, which we can read about in *Revelation 22: llll.*

01-09 [_] Well, I would say that the Perfect Foods for Mankind are the Sweet Fruits from the Tree of Life, as well as its Green Leaves, and perhaps Coconut Water to Drink, and perhaps certain Nuts, which seem to Taste Extremely Good. For Example, hardly anything on the Earth Tastes as Good as Fresh Dried Brazil Nuts, which are less than one Month Old from the Time of Harvest. However, now that Capitalism has Ruined most of Brazil, you can hardly find a Brazil Nut for Sale. Indeed, there might be 2 or 3 of them in a one-pound Can of Mixed Nuts, which Sells for 10$ or more. (I used to Buy those Cans of Mixed Nuts for only 1$, as late as 1974, and there were almost always as many as 10 Brazil Nuts in each Can, even though all of the Nuts were Roasted and Highly Salted, which was done to Work Up a Great Thirst for a Cold Beer, Coke, or some other Drink, even as the Ancient Romans sold Highly Salted Things for Working Up an Appetite for Drinks: beCause it is an Old Circus Trick for Selling Things.)

01-10 [_] So, O Elected King, if we Choose to Eat Greasy Sticky Foods — such as Hamburgers and French Fries, or Pizzas and Iced-creams — will those Foods not Lodge within our Bowels for Days, Weeks, or even Months, until the Body Digests them and Eliminates whatever the Body does not Want to Keep?

01-11 [_] Well, it is Obvious that some People have a 10-year Supply of Surplus Foods Stored Up in their Pipe Systems, as if they were Fixing to Hibernate with the Black and Brown Bears, who Fatten Up all Summer for Preparations for Long Cold Winters, when all such Bears do not Eat anything: beCause they are Designed for Hibernating, while People can Choose to Say and Do whatever they Want to: beCause we have Freedom to Do that. Therefore, we would be Wise to Choose our Eating Habits Carefully, lest we end up becoming as FAT as Walruses, and for no Sane Reasons. After all, we are Designed for Collecting Fat in our Bodies, just in Case we might have to Endure a Long Cold Winter with very little or nothing to Eat, as was the Case with the Donner Party, who became Cannibals during 1844, when they got Trapped by Capitalism, and Doomed by Ignorance, who did not know much about Fasting nor Praying, even though I am Sure that many of them did both; but, not Properly. Otherwise, they might have all Survived in Good Shape. Yes, there was a little Book written by a certain Lady who Survived a Plane Crash in Alaska, along with a certain Ignorant Man, who Attempted to Work himself to Death to Escape from it, while she simply Settled for a Long Fast, and Patiently Waited to be Rescued, while she Prayed for Help. Indeed, People have been known to Fast for YEARS on nothing but Water and Air: beCause of being Designed that Way. You can read about them in certain Books, which I have long ago forgotten the Names of: beCause of not being Able to Prove any such Things. Nevertheless, I do Agree that it is Possible to go a Long Time without Eating much of anything, if you just Relax and Rest and Forget about any Ambitions: beCause of having very Low Energy Reserves, in which Cases People could easily Survive for Long Periods of Time on just a few Gallons of Honey, IF they were Prepared for it. Yes, Honey is something that Keeps Well for a Long Time, and can be Nibbled on, a Teaspoon full at a Time, mixed with a Quart of Water or Herbal Tea. However, it is NOT a Working Man's Best Diet by any Means; but, it is only Good for Survival during Times of Famines. Such Famines are Rare, nowadays: beCause of Compassionate Governments, which usually come to the Rescue with Tons of Rancid Rice, Rancid Butter, 40-year-old Cheeses, White Flour, and perhaps Expired Canned Foods, which no one Relishes very much; but, even Rancid Butter on Stale Bread is perhaps Better than nothing, IF you are Starving to Death — except that just one Meal of it might KILL you: beCause of Lodging within your Bowels for a Lack of ROUGHAGE, which can be found in Kale Greens, Green Onions, Raw Cabbages, Lettuces, Celery, Shredded Carrots, and all Kinds of Fruits. Indeed, without the ROUGHAGE, those other Sticky Foods can simply CLOG UP your Internal Pipes, called Intestines, which are about 26 feet Long. Therefore, just Imagine HOW you might FORCE some Pizzas or Doughy Hamburgers THROUGH a Pipe that is 26 feet Long, as Opposed to Running some Watermelon through such a Pipe, which would just Naturally Drain Out by nothing more than Gravity, while those Sticky Pizzas would be COMPACTING within your Bowels, while also Causing you to BLOAT UP, if you just Ate an Apple or 2: beCause of not being Able to get on through such Clogged Up Pipes, which are Full of Greasy Sticky Undigested and Un-eliminated Ancient Foods, which only a Diarrhea could have any Profound Effects on, and only IF you were "Lucky," as they say: beCause, if you were Unlucky, you might just BLOAT UP and DIE from Eating a single Pound of Dates, while Religiously Following the Man called Moses, who Discovered Date Palms, after Wandering in the Wilderness for 40 Days or more, who somehow Crossed the Red Sea by himself, in order to get himself onto the Sinai Peninsula, which has a Gulf on each Side of it. Perhaps he Rode a Crocodile across the Sea. Whatever the Case, without Knowing for a FACT what all of the Circumstances were at that Time, if would not be Wise to make any such Miscalculations, and Eat your Last Meal of Sweet Dates after Fasting for even 20 Days: beCause they are NOT Idea Fruits for Breaking a Fast on. {See www.Amazon.com for: **"The Proper RULES for FASTING!" (The Complete Instruction Manual for True Repentance!) By The Worldwide People's Revolution!®**

01-12 [_] O Elected King, if a Person could Fast for 20 Days, and Eat a single Pound of Dates, and thus Kill himself, that seems to be any easy Way to Commit Suicide, and without Blasting one's Brains Out with a Shotgun. Moreover, I would rather Commit Suicide, than to Endure 4 Years in some Nazi Concentration Camp for Jews and Gypsies.

01-13 [_] I would rather become a Holy Man, whereby I might Transform that Recycled Sewage Water into Fresh Sweet Grape Juice, whereby I might Drink a whole Gallon of it, after going Dry for 10 Days, whereby I might Flush Out my Bowels, and thus get Rid of any Obstructions within my Bowels, and thus be Able to go on Fasting, while Living in some Cave on a Mountain with some Black Bears. However, in the Real World, neither Idea is Practical, much less Suicide by Eating Dates: beCause the Internal PAINS would be Excruciating and enough to make you Scream for Hours, if some Doctor Knife did not Quickly Operate on your Bowels, and Remove the Dates with his own Hands. However, just a couple of Tablespoons of Epson Salts mixed with a Cup of Warm Water could Save you from that Operation, and thus Save your Life. However, the Pharmacy that Sells the Epson Salts would likely be Closed by the Time that you Discovered what to Do to Save yourself; and the Medical Doctor would have no Idea where to Find any of it: beCause it would be a "Natural Remedy," which he would Naturally not Believe in, even though such Medical Doctors have been known to Administer ENEMAS, whereby the Bowels are somewhat Flushed Out from the Tail End of the Pipe System, even though the Problem might be Located in the STOMACH, which is usually what BLOATS UP! Therefore, before anyone does any Fasting, he or she should be WISE, and thus Study **"The Proper RULES for FASTING,"** which could Save his or her Life, and also Drastically Cut Down on any Future Doctor Bills: beCause, just a Moderate Amount of Fasting can Save you tens of thousands of Dollars in Doctor Bills, which no Medical Doctor would ever Mention: beCause that would be BAD for Business! Trust me, it is a Big SECRET among Medical Doctors, who also do it, themselves, when they get Violently SICK: beCause of Losing their Appetites. †§‡

01-14 [_] O Elected King of the Mountain, are you saying that True Healthcare should be FREE, and that almost all Medical Doctors should go back to School, and Learn HOW to make it Free?

01-15 [_] NO — I am NOT saying that True Healthcare should be, nor can be Free: beCause it Costs a LOT of Money to get Set Up Properly for LIVING. In Fact, each Family would Need Large Swanky Cisterns just for Water Storage, to make SURE that they have Sufficient Water for Watering dozens of Fruit Trees on no less than one Acre of Land, which each Family should have in their own **"Beautiful Swanky PALACES!" (A New Concept in Living Habits — Palaces for Poor People!) By The Worldwide People's Revolution!®** Book 066. Yes, to get Set Up Properly, we must Build those **"GLORIOUS Swanky Hotels Castles and Fortresses!" (Beautiful Planned City States for WISE Intelligent Well-Educated People with Common Sense and Good Understanding!) By The Worldwide People's Revolution!®** Book 019. Therefore, Good Healthcare is FAR from being FREE, even though it is Possible to Fast and Pray without any Money at all, if you have a True Christian Church nearby, who Practices the Teachings of Jesus Christ, who are Willing to Assist you to do the Fasting, and is also Willing to Support you with Good Sweet Unpoisoned Ripe Fruits from the Trees of Life, after Fasting, which have been Grown by: **"The LUSCIOUS All-Mineral Organic Method of Gardening!" (HOW to Grow DELICIOUS Satisfying Foods for Potential Kingz and Kweenz in Swanky PALACES!)**, Book 021, after Studying: **"Did God or Satan Ordain Medical Doctors??" (Ask Huck Finn and/or Nigger Jim: because neither Tom Sawyer nor Judge Thatcher would Know!)**, Book 022, as well as: **"The Gospel According to The Worldwide People's Revolution!®" (The Good News from the Most Modern Perspective!)**, Book 013. However, your Chances of Discovering such a Church are ZILCH: beCause there is no Major Religion in the World that Teaches what I Teach, which is a Religious Subject that most Churches want nothing to do with: beCause they like to EAT, Drink, and be Merry; but, not with Saint Mary, much less with Saint Paul, who Fasted often, according to *First ...*

01-16 [_] So, O Elected King, it Sounds as if we are up Against a SOLID Brick Wall, which is too High to get Over, too Wide to get Around, too Deep to get Under, and too Thick to Dig Through it, huh? Will Babylon have to be Overthrown, just to make it Possible for the Production of a True Church?

01-17 [_] Well, it Appears to be the Case, which is all Fair and Square with me, even if the Rain must Stop for 3 Years and 6 Months, as it is Revealed in *Revelation 11,* which Warns about it, which would be of little Effect, if it were not a Worldwide FAMINE, which it will likely be: beCause Capitalism Calls for it, having everything neatly Set Up for such a Great Famine, whereby most of the People have Forsaken the Good Land, and have Moved themselves into Cities of Confusion, whereby they are Tormented both Day and Night, who have no Idea HOW the Human Body and Mind WORKS, nor how Important it is to Eat Wholesome Natural Foods, which cannot be Found in GROSS Grocery Stores: beCause Orgimmick Gardening is NOT According to **"The LUSCIOUS All-Mineral Organic Method of Gardening,"** whereby the Plants have Access to ALL of the Necessary Minerals and Natural Fertilizers that Produce GOOD Sweet Satisfying FRUITS. Moreover, to make Matters a hundred Times WORSE, most Farmers have been a Pack of Capitalist LIES, while Filling the Skies with Poisons that come down in what they call Acid Rains from Industrialization, which Acid Rains Poison the Land and Weaken the Trees, and make them Susceptible to all Kinds of Diseases, for which Mr. Smart Farmer is Sold another Pack of Lies in the Form of Poisonous SPRAYS, which are supposed to Cure those Diseases on the Trees, much like Pain-killing Pills are supposed to Cure Arthritis and other Human Diseases — at least in the Minds of those Ignorant People who have been Deceived by Various DRUGS, which never Actually CURE anything: beCause, only the Body has the Power to Heal itself, which might be Assisted by certain Drugs or Medicines; but, once the Body has Lost its Ability to Heal itself, no Amount of MediSINZ will Cure it. Otherwise, Rich People would be the Healthiest Happiest People in the World, which they are NOT! In Fact, some of them would even like to Murder me for telling you these Things: beCause they are Related with those Ancient Scribes and Pharisees, who Orchestrated the Murder and Execution of the Most Righteous Man in the World at that Time, who may or may not have Done all of the Miracles that are Accredited to him; but, for Sure, he was Envied by those Lying Red Jews, who made up False Stories about him, even as they have made up False Stories about me. Indeed, it is Expected of them: beCause, if I am Correct, their entire Evil Empire is in Graveyard Danger of be Exposed and Deposed, which would be BAD for Business, you might say! Yes, it would be Deadly to them, even as the Teachings of Jesus Christ were Deadly to them, which is WHY the *Bible* was Carefully EDITED by them, whereby they Removed some of the most Precious Parts, including HOW to Fast, and WHY to Fast. Nevertheless, certain Information did "Sneak Through," you might say, and can still be Found in those Books — a little here, and a little there. {See www.Amazon.com for: **"Poverty Hunger Riots Strikes Brutalities Election Deceptions and Civil Wars!" (The High Price that we Earthlings have Paid for Leaving the Good Land!) By The Worldwide People's Revolution!®** Book 014.}

01-18 [_] O Elected King, we are very Thankful that you have taken the Time to Discover WHY People should FAST and PRAY: beCause it is for Sure that Medical Doctors have not taken the Time to do it, nor to even Consider it: beCause, why would they Want to put themselves OUT of Business? Therefore, in spite of the Fact that all Wild Animals have only ONE Sure Cure for whatever might Ail them, which is to Fast and Pray, those Medical Doctors are not likely to come out with a Report about the Great Benefits of Fasting nor Praying, even though a few of them have given some Credit to Praying, which even a Drunkard and Glutton can do; but, when it comes to Fasting, or Abstaining from all Foods for Long Periods of Time, that is something that very few People can Do.

01-19 [_] Well, my Friend, there are more than 100 Good Reasons WHY People should Fast and Pray, which I will List in the next Chapter for your Education, Enlightenment, and Entertainment with a little Humor: beCause it is quite Comical just HOW such "Top Secret" Information could be Hidden in the Mutilated Bible for thousands of Years, and not be Discovered by the Irreverent LOUDMOUTH Sloth-gut Windbag Hole-in-Thy-Head, who has been Preaching his Lies and Deceptions for hundreds of Years — such as that LIE about being Saved by the Grace of the Doctor Knife, whereby he might BOAST about his Good Deeds, when it is Possible and much more Practical to be Saved by the Grace of GOD, who only Requires that we Love and Obey Natural Dietary LAWS, one of which is to STOP EATING whenever we Lose our Appetites!

01-20 [_] O Elected King, Jesus said, *"He who Believes in me, not only these Wonderful Works shall he Do; but, even Greater Works — such as Transforming Rocks into Pure Gold, and Resurrecting Extinct Creatures, whereby the Earth might be Restored to its Perfect Natural Frame and Order."* — *The New MAGNIFIED Version (NMV)*

— Chapter 02 —

A List of Good Reasons WHY People Should FAST and PRAY!

02-001 [_] *"The Servant does Well to be Like his Master in all Ways."* See *Matthew 4; and 10:24—25,* in whatever Versions you Like.

02-002 [_] Holy People do not Sweat or Perspire like Unclean People, even during a Hot Day, while Fasting: beCause most of the Heat that is Generated within us comes from the Foods that are found in our Bowels. Therefore, when those Foods are Removed, we are Cool.

02-003 [_] Holy People do not get Hot while Working Hard, like Unclean People do: beCause Holy People are Slender and Stronger.

02-004 [_] Holy People do not get Cold, like Unclean People do: beCause their Blood has Better Circulation, and their Bodies Work Correctly, just like any Wild Animal, some of whom can Endure Temperatures that would Kill most People.

02-005 [_] The Mind cannot Work Correctly, until the Body is Clean on the Inside of it; and it cannot be Clean until a Person Fasts, or at least Eats very little, until his Body is Clean, which might Require Years while Eating; but, only 40 Days while Fasting and Praying, unless she is a Tub of Lard to begin with, which many People are.

02-006 [_] A Clean Body is very Beautiful after doing a lot of Fasting: beCause it becomes Youthful. (See *Jobe 33:25, KJV.*)

13

02-007 [_] You cannot be Loved, until you are Lovable; and Fasting makes you more Lovable, and Especially if you become a Holy Person, like Moses, Elijah, or Jesus, John, Peter, James, or the Apostle Paul, who *"Turned the World Upside Down."*

02-008 [_] Holy People have Power with God, *in as much as* they do Fasting and Praying and Obeying the Laws of God.

02-009 [_] Having Power with God can Result with a Blest World, if the People of the World do not Reject the Truths that you Teach, which most People will just Naturally do: because Living a Holy Life is Anti-Capitalism, which is the Love of Money in Action, which is the Root Cause for almost all Evils.

02-010 [_] All of the Holy Prophets did a lot of Fasting and Praying, and *who* would not Want to be like one of them, except for their Persecutions by Wicked People?

02-011 [_] Fasting Encourages a Person to do more Fasting, if he does Enough of it to Remove the Slime and Filth that Torments him, which can be Accumulated within Lumps, Tumors, Boils, Abscesses, Cancers, and wherever — mostly in the Lower Bowels, at the Far End of the Drainage Pipe, which some People say is the Location of the Emotions. Therefore, if someone is in a Bad Mood, that Person is likely somewhat Constipated, and Needs a Bowel Movement.

02-012 [_] Fasting can Relieve Pains: beCause the Body Naturally Produces Pain-killing Drugs while Fasting, which Explains WHY Wild Animals are not Screaming with Pains, even after getting Shot by Hunters without Consciences.

02-013 [_] Fasting and Praying is Nature's only Sure Cure, when Followed by a Natural God-given Diet, whatever it might be, which has yet to be Proven.

02-014 [_] Fasting and Praying has Healed more so-called "Incurable" Cases of Disease than any other Method of Treatment. For Example, there were more than 10,000 so-called "Incurables," who came to Professor Arnold Ehret's Fasting Sanitarium in Switzerland, during the early 1900's, and every Person who Obeyed him got Cured! I Learned that Information Personally from Fred Hirsch, who was Arnold's Assistant. (See the Internet for the **Arnold Ehret Health Club,** as well as the *Wikipedia* Article about him, which does not do him Justice.)

02-015 [_] Fasting is the Opposite of Works. Fasting is Abstaining from all Works. Indeed, it is Salvation through Faith in the Words of God, who said: *"Be you Holy, even as I am Holy, or Clean, both Inside and Outside: beCause Holiness Requires Purity of the Mind, Spirit, and Body. Therefore, except an Unclean Man should Humble himself by Means of Fasting and Praying, until he becomes like an Innocent Child with a Pure Mind and a Clean Body, he shall in no Way Enter into the Holy Kingdom of All that is Good."* (See *First Peter 1:16; and Leviticus 11:43— 45.*)

02-016 [_] *"... for without Holiness, no Man shall even See the Supreme Ruler."* — *RKJV of Hebrews 12:14.*

02-017 [_] The Greatest People who ever Lived did a lot of Fasting and Praying — such as Jesus Christ, Moses, Elijah, Isaiah, Solomon, David, Samson's Parents, Paul, Peter, John, and so on.

02-018 [_] The Best Person who ever Lived did a lot of Fasting and Praying. (See *Matthew, Mark, Luke, and John.*)

02-019 [_] Certain Demons cannot be Cast Out without a lot of Fasting and Praying. (See *Matthew 17:21, KJV.*)

02-020 [_] Fasting and Praying is the only Way to Overcome Gluttony, Drunkenness, Drug Addictions, Food Addictions, and Bad Habits that are Controlled by Internal Filth.

02-021 [_] A Person's Eyes become Clear and Bright after Fasting and Praying, which is what gives certain Ministers the Appearance of having Communed with God.

02-022 [_] I had a Heavy Red Streak in my Right Eye for 5 Years, which Disappeared after Fasting for 314 Days during 14 Months, at which Time one of Kidneys was Quivering, and then I passed out a String or "Braided" Rope-like Thing that was about as big as my little Finger, and about 8-inches long, which was a Great Relief, which gave new Meaning to the Word, Restroom.

02-023 [_] Fasting on nothing but Water will Clear up the Skin, Eyes, and Mind.

02-024 [_] Fasting and Praying makes a Person Calm, Relaxed, and Confident, and especially when he or she keep SILENT.

02-025 [_] Fasting and Praying can make a Man as Bold as a Lion, if he Persists until he is Cleaned Out.

02-026 [_] Fasting and Praying can Restore certain Organs, as well as Hair and Teeth.

02-027 [_] Fasting and Praying can make a Person Bug-resistant. That is, such Insects as Mosquitoes and Flies will not Bite a Holy Person.

02-028 [_] If a Poisonous Snake bites a Holy Person, the Poison will not Harm him. (See *Mark 16 and Acts 28.*)

02-029 [_] Fasting and Praying can make Animals be at Peace with you. Remember Daniel in the Lion's Den for the Evidence.

02-030 [_] Fasting and Praying can Save a City from Destruction. See *the Book of Jonah.* This is a Major Reason for Fasting and Praying. However, if you Want to Save your House from a Firestorm, Tornado, Hurricane, Flood, Earthquake, Mudslide, or other Natural Disaster, you have to Use WISDOM, which is a Gift from God to all People who HATE All that is Evil, who LOVE All that is Good, who Respect the Natural and Divine Laws, which Wisdom can be Gained by simply Fasting and Praying, whereby your Mind is Enlightened to some Degree, according to how much Fasting and Praying you do, combined with your Life Experiences, Nolij, and

Learning Abilities. For Example, only an Ignorant Fool would Build or Buy a House in some Swamp like New Orleans, which is Under Sea Level, where no Houses should be Built, unless they are Built on Top of Large Strong Cisterns, which are Stacked Up at least 200 feet High, just to be more Out of Reach of Ocean Tides, Hurricanes, and Floods. In other Words, it would Require a LOT of Difficult WORK to Build a Proper City in such a Swamp, which is NOT an Ideal Place to Build anything except a Delta, which Nature does for Free. So, let Nature do her Thing, as they say, and stay Out of there. However, even on the Great Plains, there are the Dangers of Wild Fires, Flood, Tornadoes, and Earthquakes. Therefore, Wise People would Work Together by United Effort to Build Fireproof, Flood-proof, Tornado-proof, Earthquake-proof, Self-air-conditioned, Rot-proof, Paint-proof, Termite-proof, Mouse-proof, and Insurance-proof Houses: so as to Prevent any Future Natural Disasters, and also Build such Cities for Self-defense, whereby Criminals and Potential Criminals can Kept Out and also Cast Out, if they are Discovered, whereby the Masses of People can Live in Peace. After all, only about 6% of the People are Psychopaths, like George Warmonger Bush and Little Dick Chicanery. Therefore, they are Welcome to Live with the Lions and Bears, Snakes and Liars, Scorpions and Poisonous Spiders in the Wilderness, along with Painted Stinking Skunks and Prostitutes.

02-031 [_] Fasting and Praying can Cause a Person to be Blest with the Gifts of God, such as the Power to do Miracles, Heal Sick People, Raise up Dead People, Transform Rocks into Pure Gold, Walk on the Water, and so on — all of which Defy Natural Laws, you might say, which is WHY they are called "Miracles": beCause those are not Natural, such as the Birth of a Baby, which seems to be quite "Miraculous" to whomever has one; but, it is not Supernatural, like People Flying about without Wings, by the Power of God.

02-032 [_] The Widow's Barrel of Flour and Cruise of Oil did not run Dry for 3 Years, after Elijah Blest her, after he took his 40-day Fast. (See *First Kings 17 and beyond.*)

02-033 [_] Fasting and Praying Saved King David from being Cursed after he Sinned. (See his own Inspired Writings for the Proof.)

02-034 [_] Fasting and Praying Saved the Jews from being Destroyed during the Days of Esther.

02-035 [_] Fasting and Praying Saved Jonah from being Digested by the Whale Shark that Swallowed him. (See *the Book of Jonah.*)

02-036 [_] Fasting and Praying Saved me from Blindness, as well as the Apostle Paul. (See *the Book of Acts 9 and 13.*)

02-037 [_] Fasting and Praying Saved all of the Men who were on the Ship that Paul was on when they were about to be Destroyed. (See *Acts 27.*)

02-038 [_] Fasting and Praying has Preceded almost all Discoveries, including that of Columbus, the Electric Light, the Telephone, the Radio, certain Television Parts, and even this Book, which would be a Great Discovery to someone whose Life was Saved by Reading it and Obeying **"The Proper RULES for FASTING!" (The Complete Instruction Manual for True Repentance!) By The Worldwide People's Revolution!®**

02-039 [_] Fasting and Praying is the single Natural Cure for all Wild Animals, who have NO Doctors, NO Drug Stores, NO Medicines, and NO Hands for Earning Money, in order to Pay for any such Vain Things: beCause they are all Healed by Fasting and Praying, alone. However, you might Argue that no Animal does any Praying: beCause of not having any Words to Pray with, even within their Minds, which is under the Assumption that they are too Stupid to Learn, which is no doubt True of some Animals, even though it can also be Argued that some Animals are much more Intelligent than People, who at least know HOW to take Advantage of the Natural Air-conditioning of the Good Earth, who Burrow into it to make their Homes Livable.

02-040 [_] Fasting and Praying makes a Mind Work so Well, that a Person can Recall Names of People and Places that he or she has Forgotten for many Years, as well as Stories that such a Person Heard many Years Ago.

02-041 [_] Fasting and Praying can Cause a Person to have Visions and Dreams concerning Important Things that are to Come, as well as New Inventions, which a Person can Visualize in his Mind — such as those **"GLORIOUS Swanky Hotels Castles and Fortresses!" (Beautiful Planned City States for WISE Intelligent Well-Educated People with Common Sense and Good Understanding!) By The Worldwide People's Revolution!®**

02-042 [_] Fasting and Praying can make a Person Feel so Good that he Wants to JUMP for JOY! (You can read about Lucy in my Inspired Book, called: **"Did God or Satan Ordain Medical Doctors??" (Ask Huck Finn and/or Nigger Jim: because neither Tom Sawyer nor Judge Thatcher would Know!) By The Worldwide People's Revolution!®**

02-043 [_] Fasting and Praying puts Fear into the Enemies, who cannot stand to Look into your Eyes: beCause they Fear that you can Read their Minds, and Know their Thoughts.

02-044 [_] Fasting and Praying is the Surest Cure for Depression, even a Guaranteed Cure!

02-045 [_] Fasting and Praying is the Surest Cure for Guilt, and the Elimination thereof, if one makes a Full Confession of all Sins, and Begs the Heavenly Father to Forgive him or her in the Name of Jesus Christ, who is the Anointed Savior, who will Forgive and Pardon almost all Sins, except for Blasphemy against the Holy Spirit, who Inspired all Good Books, including this one.

02-046 [_] Fasting and Praying can "Bend the Heart of God," and Cause him to Favor you for it. (See the Inspired Writings of Moses for the Proof.)

02-047 [_] Fasting and Praying is the only Right Thing to do when you have Lost someone whom you have Loved. (See *Genesis* for the Evidence. Remember Jacob.)

02-048 [_] If there were an Atomic Nightmare, those People who Fast and Pray might not Die from the Radiation: beCause Skinny People are not Effected much by Radiation: because the Radiation Burns the Fat in a Fat Body, which the Body cannot Eliminate before it Kills him: because it Overloads the System all at once, which is too much for the Body to Handle. Many Skinny People Survived in Hiroshima, Japan, in 1945, and also Lived to be Old.

02-049 [_] Fasting and Praying can make a Person Super Strong, so that Heavy Weights seem to be very Lightweight. This reminds me of the Time when I Fasted on Angel Ridge at King's Mountain, Kentucky, for 314 Days out of 14 Months, and after that Time, I went Outside of my House, and picked up a Heavy Limestone Rock that was 6 inches thick and about 30 inches square, and it felt as Lightweight as a little Red Brick! I would guess that it weighs more than 300 Pounds.

02-050 [_] Fasting and Praying is one of the Best Swanky Vacations that a Body can take. Therefore, Try it before you Mock it, and Do it According to **"The Proper RULES for FASTING,"** so as to be Successful with it, even if you have to Forsake everyone and everything except God to be Successful.

02-051 [_] Fasting is Nature's Operating Table, you might say, which is Free of Charge, and Free of Poisonous MediSINZ, which are Medical Sins. (It is Interesting to Note that more than 100,000 Americans Die each Year on Account of Medical "Mistakes," such as WRong Prescriptions of Drugs, or Bad Combinations of Drugs, or Drugs with Alcoholic Drinks. Therefore, Wise People would Stay Away from all Snakes with Needles and Poisons in their Heads, even as the Millions of Buffaloes used to Trample them Under their Hooves.)

02-052 [_] Fasting and Praying is much Better than lying on some Hospital Bed for MONTHS, or perhaps even for YEARS, just to be Healed from something that might be Cured within 2 Weeks — such as Arthritis, Rheumatism, and Gout. However, once a Person's Liver has been Ruined by too much Alcohol, it is Safe to say that there is no Cure Possible, even with a New Liver Implanted: beCause the Body has a Tendency to Reject Foreign Objects, including New Livers. Therefore, it is Extremely Important to STAY AWAY from Satan's Deceptive Drinks, except for perhaps a Glass of Wine at some Wedding, on Rare Occasions, as Jesus did, who even Transformed the Rainwater into Wine, just to have some more of it. Nothing was Mentioned about the Alcoholic Content of that Wine, which was likely less than 10%. However, do not use that as an Excuse for Drinking such Wine on a Daily Basis: beCause that is HOW People get Addicted to Drinking, which Naturally Calls for more and MORE, just to get what they call a "High" Feeling, which one can Obtain while Fasting, without Drinking anything! (See *John 4*.)

02-053 [_] *"You shall Learn the Truth, and the Truth shall make you Free,"* could not be any more True, than it is for the Person who Fasts and Prays, who Discovers that Great Truth about Freedom from all Accumulated Filth, Poisons, Drugs, Addictions, Pains, Headaches, Indigestion, Cramps, Bad Dreams, and all of the Evil Things that Plague Disobedient Rebellious People, who Refuse to even Experiment with Proper Eating and Proper Fasting, who never Discover that Great Truth with a Capital D, G and T. {See www.Amazon.com for: **"Justifications for Capitalizations!" (WHY The Worldwide People's Revolution!® Defies the School of Fools by Capitalizing LOVE and HATE!)** Book 049.}

02-054 [_] True Freedom can only come to the Person who Fasts and Prays: beCause he is Free Inside from all Torments of Mind, Body, and Spirit. However, the Unclean Person is Tormented both Day and Night, and Especially when he or she Weighs 200 Pounds too much.

02-055 [_] If there is one Thing that every Person should be doing before he or she Dies, it is to Fast and Pray for the Last 40 Days and 40 Nights, just to Try to Discover if God is not Right.

02-056 [_] Above all other Religious / Spiritual Experiences, none Compare with that of the Person who Fasts and Prays, until he or she is Holy in Mind, Body and Spirit, which he or she can only do by the Grace of God: beCause it is only God who makes us Holy, not ourselves. Therefore, do not Seek any Glorification for something that you have not Done; but, give all of the Glory to the Great Creator God, who alone Deserves the Honor and Glory for the Way that he Created us. Therefore, just be Thankful, and not Proud nor Boastful of it, as if you Won the Race by something that you Did to make your Muscles Strong, whereby you Deceived yourself by your own Exercises. After all, it is Possible to be much Stronger by Submitting to the Will of God, and Seeking his Divine Strength, which is much more Powerful.

02-057 [_] *"Blest are they who Patiently Wait on the Supreme Ruler by Means of Fasting and Praying: beCause they shall Renew their Strength; yes, they shall Mount Up with Wings of Great Faith, and thus be Able to Run all Day, and not be Weary, and to Walk all Night, and not Faint; but, Woe to those Foolish People, who are without Patience and Persistence, who have no Faith in the Divine Powers of the Supreme Lawmaker: beCause they shall be Spiritually Blinded by the Darkness of their own Ignorance."* — {See: **"The New MAGNIFIED Version of ISAIAH in Plain English!" (The Understandable Version of the Book of Isaiah!) By The Worldwide People's Revolution!**® Book 044.}

02-058 [_] Fasting and Praying is SUBMISSION to God, which Pleases him, unless we are doing it for Selfish Reasons. (See *Isaiah 58.*)

02-059 [_] Fasting and Praying is able to Save us from World War 3, if we Sincerely do it for Good Reasons, and Seek to Overcome all of our Sins, including our Dietary Sins, Warmongering Sins, Capitalist Sins, Pollution Sins, Worshiping Hollywood Idols, Admiring Vain Paintings, Bowing Down to False Gods — such as Capitalism, Communism, Socialism, Fascism, and Pledging Allegiance to any such Rags as the American Flag, which is Powerless to Save anyone from anything, which Satan uses to Deceive Ignorant People, and to Blind their Minds with Pride, whereby they are even Willing to Die for such Bloody Rags, rather than DEMAND **"The Great Worldwide TELEVISED Court HEARING,"** whereby they might Learn the Whole Truth about all Important Subjects, and thus put an End to all Hateful Wars, Tax Slavery, Interest Slavery, Insurance Slavery, Drug Slavery, Childcare Slavery, and Work Slavery, whereby they might be Liberated from the Prison of Lies, which they were Born into!

02-060 [_] Fasting and Praying is the only Way that a Person can Obtain "Gifts," such as a Clear Voice, which is a Normal Voice for Holy People, who can Sing like Canaries!

02-061 [_] Fasting and Praying is Frightening to People who are not Worthy to Enter into the Holy Kingdom of All that is Good, which keeps them OUT, which is very Good: beCause, who would Want to Live with Barking Dogs, Filthy Hogs, Lying Poisonous Snakes, Scorpions, Spiders, Bloodsucking Leeches, Greedy Wolves, Ravenous Lions, and Stinking Skunks?

02-062 [_] If a Person is a Coward of any Kind, he or she can be Cured by Fasting and Praying, and Especially if he or she is a Spiritual Coward, who is Afraid to Check the Boxes [_] with Statements that he or she Agrees with throughout the Literature of **The Worldwide People's Revolution!®**

02-063 [_] Fasting and Praying is the most Comforting Way to Face any Crisis, including Wars. I Know: beCause I have been there.

02-064 [_] Fasting and Praying is the Surest Way to Obtain a Natural Appetite for God-given Foods, which would not include any of the Devil's Foods, and Especially any of his Drugs.

02-065 [_] Fasting and Praying is the Spiritual Bridge that Crosses the Valley of Doubt and Fear.

02-066 [_] If there were only one Thing to Do, and you could not do anything else, it would be to Fast and Pray.

02-067 [_] If every Decision were made after Fasting and Praying about it, there would be fewer Mistakes made all around. Therefore, all Leaders should have to Fast and Pray, until they become HOLY, even as Jesus was Holy.

02-068 [_] The Best Way to begin any Day, is to Fast and Pray: beCause the Mind Works Better on an Empty Stomach, up until the Time of Elimination of Filth, or until the Body runs out of Energy, at which Time a little Honey will Solve that Problem, unless a Person is Working Hard, and Needs a LOT of Energy, in which Case Sweet Ripe Fruits Supply the Best Energy. And the next Best Things are Fresh Sweet Fruit Juices, which can keep a Body Running at Full Speed all Day Long!

02-069 [_] Fasting and Praying helps the Bowels to Work Good, and Especially if it is Combined with Weeping and Mourning for the Poor Lost Souls.

02-070 [_] If People were to Fast and Pray for 40 Days, before they go Shopping, they would Realize that almost nothing in the GROSS Grocery Stores is Fit to Eat nor Drink, whereby they might begin to get their Priorities in Order. {See www.Amazon.com for: **"HOW to Get our PRIORITIES in ORDER!" (The Glories of Democracy; and, Does DEMON-ocracy have its Priorities in Order?) By The Worldwide People's Revolution!®** Book 060.}

02-071 [_] After Fasting and Praying until your Nostrils and Taste Buds are Working Correctly, you have about as much use for the City of Pollution as you do for used Toilet Paper. But, how can you Live without all of those Vain Things — such as Polluting Cars, Lawnmowers, Garden Tillers, Tractors, Pickups, Trucks, Snow Blowers, Leaf Blowers, Snowmobiles, Motorcycles, Motor Scooters, and AIRPLANES? O Adam, how did YOU Live without all of those Vain Things? O Eve, how did you Live for 800+ Years without the million and one Vain Things that can be Found in Super Smallmart Stores? Oh, you Poor Creature! Could it be that you were Deprived of the Best Things in Life, which Caused you to Live so Long?

02-072 [_] No one would Want to get the *"Mark of the Beast,"* if they simply Fasted and Prayed for 40 Days and 40 Nights: beCause they would only Want to Live on the Land, and Raise some Fruit Trees. {See www.Amazon.com for: **"Poverty Hunger Riots Strikes Brutalities Election Deceptions and Civil Wars!" (The High Price that we Earthlings have Paid for Leaving the Good Land!) By The Worldwide People's Revolution!® Book 014.**}

02-073 [_] If you are having a Difficult Time Deciding what to Do for a Living, just Try Fasting and Praying and Meditating on: **"The Environmentalists' Paradise!" (HOW almost Everyone could be Living in a Beautiful Manmade Paradise!) By The Worldwide People's Revolution!® Book 035.**

02-074 [_] No one is so Ambitious as the Person who has just done a lot of Fasting and Praying.

02-075 [_] If you Want to Discover "New" Truths within any Inspired Book, just Try Fasting and Praying while Reading those Words more SLOWLY and Thoughtfully.

02-076 [_] Beyond Fasting and Praying, there is only one Thing that is Better, and that is more Fasting and Praying, until at Last you are Speaking with God, Face to Face on Mount Zion. {See: **"The Secret City of the Great King!" (HOW the True Church will Escape from the Great Tribulation!) By The Worldwide People's Revolution!® Book 042.**}

02-077 [_] But, before Fasting and Praying for 40 Days, do yourself a little Favor, and Fast and Pray for 4 or 5 Days on nothing but Fresh AIR; and then Flush Out your Bowels by Drinking Plenty of Fresh Fruit Juices, beginning with 2 Quarts of Fresh Immature Coconut Water; and then you will Understand WHY that I Strongly Believe in Fasting and Praying.

02-078 [_] Fasting and Praying was the "Secret" of Success that made it Possible for Kings to Conquer, as in the Case of Alexander the Great of Ancient Greece, and Adolf Hitler of Germany; and for Queens to be Accepted, as in the Case of Queen Esther and Queen Elizabeth II of Great Britain, who is still a Kindhearted Lady of Great Moderation, who is not Rolling with Lard; but, with the Lord, himself, even as her more Slender Husband has been doing for more than 94 Years.

02-079 [_] Fasting and Praying is easier than Eating and Drinking, if one has a Tendency to be a bit Lazy.

02-080 [_] Fasting and Praying is Cheaper than going to Doctors and Hospitals, and a whole lot less Expensive than Buying Groceries, if you are Broke.

02-081 [_] Fasting and Praying is like Dancing on the Head of the Devil, who will do almost anything in order to Try to get you to give it up; but, *"He who Endures unto the End shall be Saved,"* as Jesus said.

02-082 [_] Fasting and Praying is like putting the Forest Fire Out before it becomes Uncontrollable. Therefore, STOP Eating, before you are Forced to go to some Hospital, and be Humiliated by Doctors and Nurses, who Discover your Private Parts; but, not the Glory of them.

02-083 [_] The Chief Reason to Fast and Pray is to become like God, in whose Image we were Created, which cannot be Obtained without a LOT of Fasting and Praying: beCause we have Transgressed the Natural Dietary Laws, and have Removed ourselves Far from the Garden of Good Eating with a Capital F, as in Failures.

02-084 [_] Fasting and Praying makes a Person YOUNG again, even if he or she is very Old, which is called *"Regeneration"* in the *Bible.*

02-085 [_] After a Person has Fasted and Prayed, until he or she is Holy, he or she cannot Sin again: beCause the Seeds of Truths Remain within his or her Mind, in Order to Remind him or her of Right and WRong — that is, unless such an Old Person Contracts Alzheimer's Disease: beCause of Eating and Drinking from Aluminum Containers, Pots, and Pans. The Beloved Federal Government is also Busy Spraying Aluminum from Airplanes, according to the People who Study Chemtrails. (See *Wickedpedia* for the Proof.)

02-086 [_] Therefore, once a Person has Overcome all of his or her Sins, he or she is so Blest that he or she never Wants to go Back to his or her Wallowing in the Mire with the Hogs, nor Eating Vomit with the Dogs, which can Save a Person from a lot of Em-bare-assment.

02-087 [_] On the Road of Fasting and Praying, there are Humps and Bumps; but, after all of the Filth is Thoroughly Removed, the Road is as Smooth as Glass, even as Smooth as those Streets of Gold that are like Transparent Glass in the New Jerusalem.

02-088 [_] If anything will Inspire the People of the World to Fast and Pray, it will be one Holy Man, who has Obtained the Gift of God to Raise Up the Woolly Mammoth Elephants from his own Garden.

02-089 [_] Fasting and Praying is not Desirable for those People who are already Healthy, unless they come to Realize that Fasting and Praying can make them even more Healthier; and a LOT of Fasting and Praying can make them Unbelievably Healthy and Strong, such as Samson Experienced in all of its Glory.

02-090 [_] Fasting and Praying is the Last Resort for Fools, who are Forced by Famines and Wars to GIVE UP and QUIT; but, for Wise People, Fasting and Praying is the First Resort: because, *"It is more Blest to Give, than to Receive."* And Fasting and Praying are like Giving in to what God Wants; but, Eating and Drinking are like Getting what God does not Want.

02-091 [_] Fasting and Praying are Better than Partying and making a Fool of yourself for the Glory of Satan, who could care less if you went to Hell on Greased Roller-skates, or on Empty Beer Bottles.

02-092 [_] Fasting and Praying seems to be Difficult, until you get Rid of the Acids and Gasses in the Bowels, and then it becomes more Difficult to Resist your Worldly Ambitions, which can Consume all of your Thoughts, and at Last Destroy your Soul. Therefore, GIVE UP those Worldly Ambitions, until you Overcome all of your Sins, and Obtain the Superior Gifts of the Supreme Ruler, who will Provide an Abundance of whatever you Need to Succeed, after that.

02-093 [_] When you Doubt whether or not God Exists, just Try Doing what he Commanded you to Do, and Begin by Fasting and Praying, which will Result with Great Faith in him, and much less Confidence in Weak-minded People, who cannot even Agree to Work Together with United Effort for Accomplishing Great Things — such as Constructing those **"GLORIOUS Swanky Hotels Castles and Fortresses,"** which have no less than 5,000 Advantages over Normal Cities of Confusion!

02-094 [_] Before you Judge and Condemn Fasting and Praying, you should Try Doing it According to **"The Proper RULES for FASTING!" (The Complete Instruction Manual for True Repentance!)**: beCause I am Living Proof that Fasting and Praying are GOOD Habits for us to get into.

02-095 [_] There is only one Thing that is more Enjoyable than Fasting and Praying, and that is to Endure Enough of it, until you are the Healthiest Happiest Person that you know! But, of course, even then, some Capitalist Warmonger can Murder you in the Name of some False God, and Sincerely Believe that he has done God some Great Service, which he would have had a very Difficult Time Doing, if you had been Living in some Well-Fortified Planned City State — such as one of those **"GLORIOUS Swanky Hotels Castles and Fortresses!" (Beautiful Planned City States for WISE Intelligent Well-Educated People with Common Sense and Good Understanding!) By The Worldwide People's Revolution!®** Book 019.

02-096 [_] Rather than go to War over the Last Loaf of Stale Bread, or over the Last Cup of Recycled Sewage Water, it would be much Better to Fast and Pray; and, if that does not Work, it is Better to Surrender to the Enemy, and Cheerfully Cooperate, rather than be Destroyed for Pride and Foolishness: beCause, …

02-097 [_] while Fasting and Praying for your Enemies, they can be Humbled unto the Dust!

02-098 [_] If you Fear the Captivity of the Enemy, who might Conquer you, you might Want to Consider the Fact that most Enemies have put their Prisoners on Fasts, and have Forced them to go Hungry: beCause they are usually Poor and Hungry, themselves. Therefore, before God Delivers you over to the Enemies, in Order to Learn about Fasting, and perhaps in a most Difficult Way, it is Wiser to do it where you have lots of Fresh Sweet Fruits, Fruit Juices, and whatever you Want and/or Need to do it with Comfort, rather than wait until you are Imprisoned like Harlan Popov, who wrote: *Tortured for his Faith,* which is one very Sad Story with an even Sadder Conclusion: beCause, even after Experiencing all of that Fasting and Starvation, he did not come to Realize what was Required to become a Holy Man!

02-099 [_] Even if you like to Fast and Pray, it is no Fun if you are in some Prison Camp: beCause the Beds are usually Hard, and the Foods are not Fit to Eat, much less to Break a Fast on. Therefore, it is Wise to do your Fasting and Praying at a Swanky Fasting Sanitarium, if you cannot Manage yourself at Home. (FOOTNOTE: A Swanky Fasting Sanitarium is a Place where you Commit your Body to those People whom you can Trust to do what is Right for you; and therefore, you are Willingly and Voluntarily Forced to Fast for your own Good; but, a Swanky Institution of Correction is a Place where you are Forced to Fast, even if it is Against your own Will, which is Imposed onto you by some Government, which can be Good or Bad.)

02-100 [_] After Fasting for several Days, you might Appear to be Sickly and Pale; but, you can be Comforted by the Fact that before every Tree Blossoms during the Springtime of a New Birth, all of the Old Leaves Fade and Fall Off, which, to some People, Appears to be the Death of them; but, we who have Good Memories, Know that it is just a Lifecycle and a Natural Thing, which is not to be Feared. Therefore, have Faith in the God of Regenerations and Resurrections, and Trust him to take Good Care of you while Fasting and Praying according to **"The Proper RULES for FASTING,"** which are a Bit Difficult; but, nothing like a Horse Cure, which is to Fast with nothing to Eat nor Drink, until you are either Healed or Dead!

02-101 [_] Fasting and Praying are not so Dangerous, if you Remember to Follow **"The Proper RULES for FASTING!" (The Complete Instruction Manual for True Repentance!) By The Worldwide People's Revolution!®**, Book 046. However, whomever Disobeys those Rules is likely to get himself into BIG Trouble — as in a Bloated Belly, which might even Kill him, or at least Greatly Discourage him from Doing it again, which is the Equivalent of Death, itself: beCause such a Person can Die a Spiritual Death, becoming Dead to All that is GOOD. Therefore, before you Fast, you must Learn HOW to do it Correctly: because it is Possible to Kill yourself by your own Ignorance, and Especially if you already Imagine that you Know all that you Need to Learn about it, which is like a Child Attempting to Build a Stone Castle, without any Experience, and without any Teacher, which he is Unlikely to Accomplish.

02-102 [_] There is a Way that seems to be Right to People who have the Appetites of Hogs and Dogs; but, the End thereof is the Way of Sickness, Disease, and Death: beCause they do not do Enough Fasting nor Praying, whereby their Minds might be Enlightened, whereby they might have what is called "Good Judgment," whereby they might make Riit Disizhunz.

02-103 [_] Moses went up onto a Desert Mountain, in Order to do his Fasting and Praying: beCause it has its own Great Advantages. First of all, there is nothing there to Eat, so there is nothing to Tempt you to Eat it. Secondly, it is Difficult to leave such a Place until you are Strong Enough to do it, which is after the Filth has been Eliminated from your Body, which might Require 30 to 40 or more Days. Thirdly, it is a Clean Quiet Place, where you can Cry with Freedom, Knowing that only God is Listening. Fourthly, if you do manage to Overcome your Lusts, the Holy Angels are more likely to Visit with you, and even Feed to you Fresh Fruits from Mount Zion. (See *Deuteronomy 9:9 and 18; plus Matthew 4.*)

02-104 [_] Some People look on Fasting and Praying as a thing for Sissies; but, the Truth is just the Opposite — it Requires a Real Man or True Wombman to do very much Fasting and Praying; and it Requires more than a Man to Conquer the Devil, as in the Case of Jesus Christ, who was the Chief Example of Holy Men, even though he was also God, which Means that he was Chosen to be the Supreme Ruler of this World: beCause of Passing Spiritual and Physical Tests in other Worlds of Higher Orders. After all, this World is one of the Lowest and Meanest of all Worlds, which is Infested with many Unwanted Creatures, most of which were Transported here from other Mean Worlds, which will one Glad Day be Removed from the Earth when it is Cleansed by DEVOURING FIRE! Indeed, God is not going to have his Holy Angels Baby-sitting Atomic Abominations for Eternity.

02-105 [_] Fasting and Praying is not very Popular among Gluttons nor Drunkards; but, it is still more Popular among them than it is among Liars and Hypocrites, who do not Confess that it is Worse to be a Liar, than to be a Glutton: beCause a Weakness of the Mind is Worse than a Weakness of the Body. Nevertheless, the Glutton probably has some Weakness of the Mind, which Causes him to be what he is, which is very Humiliating: beCause his Sins are so Obvious, whereas the Sins of the Liar might not be so Obvious. However, since there is nothing Secret with God, everyone gets his or her Just Reward, and Especially those People who Fast and Pray, whose Reward is Strength of Character.

02-106 [_] There are probably a thousand Good Reasons to Fast and Pray, or even a million Reasons; but, whoever has to have any Reason, other than the Fact that God COMMANDED IT, is likely to Fail: beCause, without a certain Fear of God in the Bones, a Man can hardly Do what he Knows to Do: beCause Reason and Logic are Overcome by Circumstances, Hunger, Lusts, Temptations, Fears of Starving to Death, Fears of Losing one's Boring Job, Fears of being Mocked, Fears of Failing to Succeed, and so on. Therefore, by the Fear and/or Love of God, it is Possible to Fast and Pray until all Fears Vanish, and you are then Ready for the Lion's Den, or even for the Fiery Furnace of the Great Tribulation, which will be Seven Times as HOT as any other Tribulation!

02-107 [_] Before you Despair of any Hope for Fasting and Praying, just consider how many thousands of People Succeeded with it, and some are still Alive after thousands of Years! (See *John 21 and the Stories of Enoch and Elijah.*)

02-108 [_] Nothing in the Public Library, nor on Television, is as Enlightening to the Mind as Fasting and Praying for 40 Days and 40 Consecutive Nights; but, who has Time to do it while Trying to Pay all of the Bills? Truly, only the Liberated People have Time to Do it, and all of the others are Prisoners of Societies, who have no Idea what it Means to be Free with a Capital F. Therefore, Join Forces with others who are Doing it, and Pool your Resources: so that at least some of you might Succeed.

02-109 [_] The Surest Cure for Impotence, or Erectus Disfunctionus, is to Fast and Pray. Moreover, you will not Need nor Want Viagra, a Cock Ring, nor a Penis Pump, in Order to Maintain an Erection for 4 Hours, or even for 8 Hours, if you Want it; but, I have no Idea WHY you would Want it, unless you just Happen to have a 9.5-inch-long Ding Dong: beCause of Fasting and Abstaining from Sex when you were 12 to 20 Years Old, which will Actually Produce much larger Testicles than Normal, if you are a Moderate Working Person, which Large Testicles will Naturally Stimulate HARD Erectus Functionus, Nightly, while you Sleep, which will also Cause your Penis Muscles to Grow Larger, and Especially IF you Abstain from Masturbating very much until you are 18 or so, at which Time you could get Married, and not Masturbate yourself at all. However, if you are Tormented by it, Fasting will Diminish your Sperm and Seminal Fluids, if you do Enough Fasting, whereby you never have to Masturbate; but, Resisting the Pleasure of it will then become your Greatest Temptation: beCause that Sensual Pleasure is Greatly Enhanced by Means of Fasting.

02-110 [_] Fasting and Praying will not only Shrink your Stomach; but, it will Enlarge your Brains — both Left and Right — which has a Double Advantage among a hundred others.

25

02-111 [_] If you do Enough Fasting and Praying, you can Read Minds, and Sense almost everything that is about to Happen to you, in Advance. (However, that can Prove to be both Good or Bad, depending on what it is. It is called "Premonition." For Example, I have a Premonition that a Great Atomic Nightmare will Occur, if People do not Do some Fasting and Praying, until they come to Realize the Need for: **"The Great Worldwide TELEVISED Court HEARING!"** Therefore, I Strongly Recommend that all Righteous People should FLEE from all Major Cities of Confusion, and Especially New Yuck City: beCause it Contains the Chief Criminals, who are Identified as Lying Red JEWS, who Control the Money Supply, who are in Charge of the Military Industrial Congressional News Media Bankers' COMPLEX that former President Dwight David Eisenhower Warned us about in his Final Speech.)

02-112 [_] After Fasting and Praying, you need less Sleep. For Example, it is now 3:19 A.M., and I have Watched at least a dozen Educational Programs while also writing this Book, Today.

02-113 [_] If you have Trouble Sleeping, all you have to do is Enough Fasting and Praying, until at Last you can Sleep like a Baby all Night — that is, IF you have Innocent Child-like Thoughts.

02-114 [_] Fasting makes it possible to Forget about Shopping, Cooking, Eating, Washing Dishes, Drying Dishes, and all that Torments the Person who is Preparing a Feast, and then Cleaning Up after the Feast, which they Hate the most.

02-115 [_] Fasting is Condemned by Uneducated People — some of whom consider themselves to be Experts — who have never Practiced Fasting According to **"The Proper RULES for FASTING!"** However, they have only drawn up Irrational Conclusions upon their own Blundering Mistakes, which is Exactly what they Deserve, along with all of their Aches and Pains and Pills and Doctor Bills: beCause they have Spoken Evil of that which is Very GOOD — such as those **"GLORIOUS Swanky Hotels Castles and Fortresses,"** which just Happen to have more than 5,000 Good Reasons and Great Advantages for Building them and Living within the Borders of them, which nothing else on the whole Earth can Compete with for Great Advantages. Moreover, it is also a Great Advantage for them to Mock it: because it keeps People from being Eternally Damned for Rejecting Truths without any Justifiable Causes — even though their Cause is False, it is still a Cause within their own Minds, which Liberates them from any Condemnation for that Subject.

02-116 [_] Fasting makes it Possible to get the True Flavors of whatever you are Eating, or even Smelling of. No Wild Mammals will Eat anything without Smelling of it, first, and a Hungry Horse will not even Eat a Watermelon Rind, unless it is Grown by **"The LUSCIOUS All-Mineral Organic Method of Gardening!" (HOW to Grow DELICIOUS Satisfying Foods for Potential Kingz and Kweenz in Swanky PALACES!) By The Worldwide People's Revolution!®** Book 021. However, a Cow will Eat just about any Kind of Vegetation, even if it is Grown by Harmful Chemicals, Pesticides, Herbicides, and whatever, which may also form Tumors within her Body: beCause of not being Discrete with her Diet. Therefore, Cows are often Fed Absurd Foods — such as Chicken Litter, which has a Base of Sawdust. Therefore, the next Time you Bite into a Beefsteak, just Consider what all you might be Ingesting.

02-117 [_] Just the Smell of a Barnyard, after Fasting for a couple of Weeks, would Turn Off any Aware Person, and make him or her Want to RUN from it. However, it is still a very Pleasant Smell, when Compared with a Chemical Factory, or even the Smell of some RAAD, or other Pesticide, which should be Against the Law to Sell it. The Best Way to keep the Bugs OUT of your House, and everyone else's House, is to put MOATS around them with Running Water. One of my Books tells just HOW to do that Properly; but, I am Sorry that I have Forgotten the Name of it, and do not have my Master Index Constructed as of this Date. It is possibly Explained in: **"A Sound Argument for Masters and Servants!" (WHY Everyone Needs a Good Master, and every Master Needs Good Obedient Servants!)**; Book 008, or, **"WHY are some Preachers so POOR?" (HOW almost all Preachers could Get RICH, without Preaching any Outlandish LIES!) By The Worldwide People's Revolution!®** Book 009.

02-118 [_] If you Want to Discover the True Flavor of Milk, you should take one Tablespoon full into your Mouth, and Hold it there for 5 Minutes, while taking Notice of the Flavor of it, which gets Worse and WORSE as it stays in your Mouth. This will be a True Scientific Test, which any Person can do at Home for less than a Penny — that is, IF such a Person is Brave Enough to Do it. And that also Explains WHY many People Camouflage their Milk by adding Sugar, Chocolate, or something else to it — such as their Cereal for Breakfast, which is usually Loaded with Refined White Sugar.

02-119 [_] Now, as you have probably Concluded for yourself — that Fasting and Praying is the ONE and ONLY "CURE-ALL" Remedy that is Known to Mankind — so too will other Wise People Discover it by Doing it, whereby you might Save their Souls from a lot of Suffering, just by Setting a Good Example for them to Follow. After all, there is hardly a Physical, Mental, nor Spiritual Problem that it will not Solve: beCause, while Fasting and Praying, the Mind gets itself into the Right Order; and therefore, it can figure out HOW to Solve all of the other Problems.

02-120 [_] For Example, it was during a 40-day Coconut Water Fast in Hawaii, during 1980, when I first had it Revealed to me about the Goodness of Swanky Fortresses; but, it Required 10 more Years of Fasting and Praying, before I Decided to Write a Book about those hundreds and thousands of Advantages for Building such Fortresses: beCause, when it was first Revealed to me, I was not a True Believer: beCause of not Realizing what is Required for becoming a Holy Man. Nevertheless, everyone in the World can now Thank God that I did not give up on Fasting and Praying.

— Chapter 03 —

What IS a Holy Man?

03-01 [_] Well, first of all, I want to make it Clear that there is a Good Chance that I have never Actually Met a Holy Man, except for Jesus Christ, himself, and another Person who Miraculously Appeared to me while I was taking a Shower in Vietnam, who also Miraculously Disappeared. And then, about 50 Years ago, I happened to be in the Desert, near Death Valley, in Nevada, and just happened to meet a tall Young Man who came off of a 40-day Fast, who had no Idea what Foods were Proper for Breaking such a Long Fast, who Fell Headlong into an All-you-can-Eat "Free" Buffet, which had mostly Macaroni and Cheese Dishes, and no Fruits at all; but, it did not Stop him from Eating. He was Accompanied by 4 Women — all of whom were into some "Hippy Trip," as some called it. Nevertheless, he was Unbearable to Look at: beCause his Eyes and Skin were so Clear. I was actually Afraid to Speak to him, which was also True for the Man in the Shower Room. Howbeit, Dr. Springer, who was about 80 Years Old, said that he had never Seen a Healthier Person during his entire Life than myself; and therefore, he Wondered WHY I Wanted to Fast at his Resort in the Desert? Of course, I did not tell him that I Wanted to become a Holy Man, like Moses nor Elijah; but, that was what I was Aiming at, and, of course, I did not Succeed: beCause I did not have the Proper Foods to Eat after Fasting. Indeed, I was Caught in the same Capitalist Confusion that those other People were Caught in.

03-02 [_] O Elected King, could you not Find anyone to Help you? Was there no Church of God anywhere around?

03-03 [_] Well, there were Plenty of Churches of Satan all around, and in almost every City that I went to from Coast to Coast; but, as for any Churches of God, I Failed to Discover any. In Fact, it was as if I was not Supposed to Discover any: beCause they might have Messed Up my Mind with their False Doctrines — one of which was, "You cannot be Saved by Fasting and Praying," which Inspired me to say: "Well, if that is True, HOW were the People of Nineveh Saved?" And all Minds would go Blank. However, if some did not go Blank, they did after reading *Matthew 12:41*. {Please Check up on it for yourself. See also *the Book of Jonah* for the Rest of the Story, which I have MAGNIFIED in: **"The Gospel According to The Worldwide People's Revolution!®" (The Good News from the Most Modern Perspective!)**, which is in Line with the Teachings of Jesus Christ.}

03-04 [_] O Elected King, if after 50 Years or more of Fasting and Praying, you have not Managed to become a Holy Man, yourself, it could be that you have a WRong Definition of a Holy Man. Indeed, you Sincerely Believe that a Holy Man must be Pure in Mind, Spirit, and Body, which is NOT a Biblical Definition: beCause those so-called "Holy Men" were Eating whatever was Set in front of them, including Pork, Shrimps, Snails, Slugs, and Boiled Leeches! After all, *"It is not that which Enters into a Man's Mouth that Defiles him; but, it is that which come Out of his Mouth, which comes from his Heart, which is Full of Lusts, Greed, Selfishness and Backbiting."* Indeed, you Speak Evil of those Holy Churches, yourself, which is BAD: beCause they are GOOD God-fearing People, who only Curse and Use God's Name in Vain when they go to Work, and Discover that they are Ignorant People, who do not know HOW to Work without Cursing: beCause they do not Feel like Working. Therefore, almost every Move they make is WRong, which makes them Angry and Full of Cursings — such as "Damn this," and "to Hell with that!" Indeed, they only Wear Religious Masks when they Attend Church Services: beCause they are First Class Hypocrites! Moreover, if you Cross them, they are likely to Kill you for it: beCause they are Related with those Ancient Scribes and Pharisees that Jesus had to Contend with.

03-05 [_] Well, they come in all Kinds and Colors; but, the Worst of them are the Pentecostal Hypocrites, as far as I have Discovered, who even Profess to Believe in Fasting and Praying, who are less like Christ than Satan, himself, in some Cases, who will say and do just about anything **"For the Love of Money!"** And their Heels are quickly followed by the Mormons and other Moneygrubbers, who seem to be Able to Overlook their own Books: beCause it is all just a Religious SHOW, and a Big PRETENCE that they are Holy, when they Obviously have no Idea what it Means to be Holy in any Way.

03-06 [_] So, O Elected King, it seems that your Inspired Books Seek for a Way to make it Practical for almost everyone to become a Holy Person, which seems to be very Unrealistic to me: beCause it is something that hardly anyone is Seeking, and for several Good Reasons. First of all, there is no one to Inspired them to become Holy: beCause such a Person would have to Do Miracles, just to get their Attention. Secondly, such a Person would have to Live the Life of Christ, which is one of Extreme Poverty: beCause it is more Difficult for a Rich Person to Enter into the Holy Kingdom of All that is Good, than for a Camel to pass through the Gate called "the Eye of the Needle," which was a Gate on a Wall going around Jerusalem, which was left Open at Night, whereby Travelers could get into the City, if their Camels could pass through the Eye of the Needle, which Required that all such Camels had to be Unloaded, and then get down on their Knees and Crawl through the Opening, which was easy to Guard: beCause only one such Camel could squeeze through the Hole, and only if he was not too Fat. Therefore, it was Extremely Difficult for those Camels to get through the Gate, which Jesus was Comparing to the Difficulty of a Rich Man getting into the Kingdom of God with all of his Luggage and Worldly Possessions and whatever he might Want to Drag along with him for Security. Indeed, the Visitor had to pass all of his Belongings through the Eye of the Needle, first, along with any Weapons, before the Camel could pass through it, which was as good as being Strip Searched: beCause, while the Camel was Struggling to get through the Hole, all such Belongings were being Searched by the Guards, who wrote down an Inventory of such Belongings, just to make Sure that such a Person could be Held Accountable for whatever he Departed from the City with, which had to have a Receipt for every Purchase, before he could get Out. Otherwise, it was Presumed that he Stole it. Indeed, even if he Traded something that he brought into the City, for something that he Wanted, other than Foods and Drinks, he had to have a Receipt that Revealing it, whereby he could be Taxed for it: beCause he was a Foreigner, who had to Pay the Price for Visiting the "Holy City," which had its own Corruptions from Time to Time, Depending on WHO was in Charge of it. ‡

03-07 [_] Well, I would not Know all about that; but, it Sounds Reasonable enough to Believe it: beCause that would be something that Red Jews would do for Visitors, who probably got Robbed more than once at "the Eye of the Needle." Indeed, they were likely Taxed as they Entered in, just to make Sure that those Jews got their "Fair Share" of whatever someone else

Earned by Hard Labor. After all, they were the Unholy Ones who Set Up such an Evil System, and have Maintained it ever since then, even though no such System was ever Needed, nor Wanted by the Masses of People, who are now Tax Slaves, Interest Slaves, Insurance Slaves, Drug Slaves, Debt Slaves, Childcare Slaves, Social Insecurity Slaves, ElecTrickery Slaves, and Work Slaves, whose Houses are Designed for Eternal Heating and Cooling Bills, even though the Good Earth Offers it for Free, in Exchange for a little Work by some Mechanical Beasts — such as those Backhoes, Bulldozers, Trains, Concrete Mixers, and Cement Factories.

03-08 [_] O Elected King, what you are saying is that someone would have to be in Charge of this World, other than Satan and Sons, Incorporated, whose only Interest is in making SLAVES of the Masses of People, whereby no one is even Free to become a Holy Man, unless he can figure out how to Live in the Wilderness with John the Baptist, which is not a very Glamorous Lifestyle. Indeed, everyone in the World should be Free to become Holy, if they Want to; but, with the Present Arrangement of Things, that is an Impossibility for the Masses of People.

03-09 [_] Well, I must Agree with you, and I also Trust that most People will Check the above Box with an X: beCause they also Agree with you. However, if anyone Vainly Imagines that they can become Holy, even as Jesus was Holy, or as Moses was Holy, and without the Assistance of other People, let them have at it, as they say. Yes, let them Prove it by Doing it.

03-10 [_] O Elected King, there must be many *Scriptures* that Deal with such an Important Subject as this, which would also Reveal HOW to Accomplish Holiness without Selling all that we have, and Distributing the Money among Poor People, as you have done, and as Jesus did. Indeed, there must be a Way to Win this Game without becoming Poor Miserable Beggars on the Streets of Cities of Confusion.

— Chapter 04 —

Scriptures that Pertain to Becoming Holy

04-001 [_] I have Hidden your Inspired Words of Divine Truths within my Heart: so that I might Remember them, and thus not Sin against you, O Master Farmer. — Psalm 119:11, NMV.

04-002 [_] I Humbled my Soul by Means of Fasting and Praying … Psalm 35:13, RKJV.

04-003 [_] Except an Unclean Man should Humble himself by Means of Fasting and Praying, until he becomes like an Innocent Child with a Pure Mind and a Clean Body, both Inside and Outside, he shall in no Way Enter into the Holy Kingdom of All that is Good: beCause no Unclean Thing will Enter into it, lest it should Defile it. Indeed, you must become Holy, even as I, the Supreme Ruler, am Holy: beCause, without Holiness, no Person shall See my Face. — The NMV. (See *Mark 8:34; Matthew 16:24—28; and ...*

04-004 [_] My Neez are Weak from Fasting, and my Flesh Fails of any Fatness: because I am just Skin and Bones for the most part; but, I am still Alive and Able to Think Well. — NMV. (See *Psalm 109:24.*)

04-005 [_] Therefore, also NOW, says the Supreme Ruler, Turn you even to me with all of your Heart — by Means of Fasting, and with Weeping and Mourning — yes, Tear your Hearts away from the Evil Addictions that Torment the Hardhearted Rebels, whose Necks are STIFF with PRIDE, who are Dancing at their own Funerals; and do not bother to Tear your Clothing: because Torn Clothing will not Heal your Soul, nor Restore the Truth and Wisdom to Guilty Consciences; and thus Turn to the Great Creator God, who is your Supreme Ruler and Divine Lawmaker: because he is Gracious and Merciful, slow to get Angry, and of Great Kindness, who Turns himself Away from the Evil that he has Determined to Do to those People who are Evil, if they Confess their Sins, and Repent of all of their Wickedness. — NMV. (See *Joel 2:12.*)

04-006 [_] Be you not Unequally Yoked Together with Unbelievers, even as no Good Farmer would Plow with an Ox and an Ass Together: because it is Confusion. Indeed, what Fellowship is there between Righteousness and Unrighteousness? Moreover, what Communion does Light have with Darkness? And what Concord does Christ have with the Devil? Or, what Inheritance does a Believer have with an Infidel? And what Agreement does the Temple of God have with Idols, seeing that your Bodies and Minds are the Temple of the Living God, whereby your Minds are the Holiest Places within the Temple, which is called the Holy of Holies, even as God has said in Times Past: *"I will Live within them, and will Walk with them, and will Talk with their Spirits; and therefore, I will be their Supreme Ruler, and they will be my Humble, Chosen and Obedient People."* Therefore, he now says, "Come Out from among those Wicked Ones, and be you Separated from them, says the Divine Ruler, and do not Touch any of their Unclean Things; and then I will Receive you, and will be a Loving Father unto you, and you shall be my Holy Sons and Purified Daughters, says the Almighty God." Therefore, having those Good Promises, dearly Beloved Brothers and Sisters — that God will Walk with us and Give to us his Holy Spirit

— let us Cleanse ourselves from all Filthiness of the Flesh and Spirit, by Means of Fasting and Praying, while Perfecting our Holiness in the Fear and Reverence of the Supreme Ruler, who is well Able to Cast us Down into the Lowest Hellish Condition in this World, or even into a World of a Lower Order, which is Seven Times more Evil than this World; or otherwise to Raise us Up to Thrones of Glory within his Holy Kingdom, whose Worlds are Multiplying like the Birds of the Sky and the Fishes of the Seas, even Worlds without any End. Amen. — NMV. (See *Second Corinthians 6:14—7:1, KJV.*)

04-007 [_] WHAT? — do you not Know that your Mind and Body is the Temple of the Living God, and that the Spirit of God should Live within you, if you are Holy, even as he is Holy? Therefore, if any Man Knowingly, Deliberately, and Persistently Defiles the Temple of God, him shall God Destroy: beCause the Temple of God is a Holy Place, which must not be Defiled with WRong Thoughts, Drugs, Poisons, nor with WRong Foods, which were not Designed to be Eaten by People, even as People were not Designed to Eat any such Foods: beCause each Creature is Designed to Eat certain Foods, which you can Discover by Observing the Wild Animals. Moreover, you now Know that the Spirit of God does not Live in Unclean Temples, the same as you do not have any Desire to Live in a Filthy House: because it is Repulsive to you. Therefore, if your Mind and Body are not Clean, you Know that the Clean Spirit of the Supreme Ruler will not Live within you. Therefore, let no Man Deceive himself by any Means — Thinking that God will Save him in his Sins, while he is Living in a State of Filthiness — because no Unclean Thing shall Enter into the Holy Kingdom of All that is Good. Therefore, if any Man among you seems to be Wise in this World, let him become a Fool in the Eyes of the Worldly-minded People, so that he can be Truly Wise: because the wisdom of the People of this World, along with all of their Drugs and Poisons and Medicines, is utter Foolishness with the Supreme Ruler, who made every Body on this Earth to Heal itself, without the Assistance of Drugs nor Poisons of any Kind. Indeed, it is written, *"He Traps the Worldly-wise People with their own Craftiness, and brings to nothing the so-called Nolij of the Proud Fools, who Reject the Greater Counsel."* And again it reads, *"The Lord Knows the Thoughts of the Worldly-wise People, that their Thoughts are all in Vain."* Therefore, let no Man Glory in the wisdom of the Children of Unclean Men: because their Thoughts and Deeds will PERISH — but, the Thoughts and Deeds of the Holy Ones shall Endure the Test of Time. Indeed, all of the Good Words and Good Deeds of everyone is our Inheritance — whether or not they come from Paul, Apollos, Cephas, James, John, Moses, or even from the Men of the World, who have Written many Inspired Books for our Learning, even concerning Things of Life and Death, or of Things that are Present, or of Things that are to Come — all are yours, and you are Christ's, and Christ is God's Good Gift to the World, who Set a Good Example for us to Follow. — NMV. (See *First Corinthians 3:16—23.*)

04-008 [_] And David said: "Let their Dining Tables be made like Snares, Stumbling Blocks, and Traps, even Places where they are Repaid for their Lusts. Let their Eyes be Blinded by Pride, whereby they cannot See the Light of Truths, unless they Repent of their Evil Ways, Perverse Thoughts, and Wicked Deeds: so that they are Blinded to the Riit Waa: so that they might not See the one and only Way Out of their Self-dug Pit of Self-destruction; and may they Bow Down their Backs forever in the Fields of the Devil, being Slaves of Sins, and Prisoners of Lies." — NMV. (See *Romans 11:9—10.*)

04-009 [_] Have you not Learned anything about the Holy Ones? Have you not Heard that the Everlasting Supreme Ruler, who Lives in Glorious Mansions in the Heavens, who has Allowed Satan to Tempt and Test our Spirits, and to Rule Over this World, is the Creator of Endless Worlds, and the Creator of every Good Thing in this World, even unto the Ends of the Earth, does not Faint, neither is he Weary after Working all Day? There is no Searching Out the Extent of his Good Understanding nor Wisdom. He Gives Power to the Weak People, who Submit to his Will; and to those who have no Might, he Increases their Strength beyond Belief. Yes, even the Youthful Children shall Faint and be Weary, and the Young Men shall utterly Fall; but, they who Patiently Wait on the Supreme Ruler by Means of Fasting and Praying, shall Renew their Strength — they shall Mount Up with Wings of Great Faith, like the Eagles, you might say; they shall Run all Day Long, and not be Weary; and they shall Walk all Night Long, and not Faint. — NMV. (See *Isaiah 40:28—31.*)

04-010 [_] Bless the Supreme Ruler, O my Soul, and all that is within me, Bless his Holy Name. Bless the Anointed Savior, O my Soul, and do not Forget any of his Great Benefits. Indeed, he Forgives all of our Iniquities, if we Beg him to; and he Heals all of our Diseases, if we Cooperate with his Laws of Nature; yes, he Redeems our Lives from the Pit of Self-destruction, he Crowns us with Loving Kindness and Tender Mercies, and he Satisfies our Mouths with Good Sweet Fruits: so that our Youthfulness is Renewed like that of the Eagle's Youth, who gets New Feathers, and one at a Time: because it is the Process of Regeneration, which Requires Time while Fasting and Praying. Therefore, be Patient, be Bold, be Brave, be Strong, and Endure unto the End, until you have Overcome all of the Filthiness within your Mind and Bowels, where it Lodges in the Unclean Person. — NMV. (See *Psalm 103:1—5.*)

04-011 [_] For God Speaks once — yes, sometimes TWICE, even during the same Day — and yet Evil Men do not Perceive it. In a Dream, in a Vision of the Night — when Deep Sleep falls on Men, in Slumberings upon their Beds — then the Supreme Ruler Opens the Inner Ears of Men, and Seals their Instructions in their Minds: so that he might Withdraw Men from their Evil Works, and also Hide Pride from them: because the Spirit of Pride is the most Blinding Force of Self-destruction in the World, which is also used to get Foolish Men to go to War, and Sacrifice their Lives in Vain, when it is Possible and most Practical for all People to be Living within the Borders of Beautiful Fortresses, which are Designed for Living, even as the Garden of Eden is Designed for Perfect Peace, which is Hidden in the Secret Place of the Most High Ruler. Yes, the Supreme Ruler keeps back the Humble Soul from Falling into the Pit of Self-destruction, and also Saves his Life from Perishing by the Sword of Revenge in any War. He is Corrected also with Pains while lying on his own Bed of Sorrows, and the Multitude of his Bones are Affected with TERRIBLE Pains: so that his Body Abhors Foods of all Kinds, except Fresh Fruit Juices; and his Spirit Detests Dainty Foods, and especially Greasy Sticky Foods, which Act like Glue within his Pipe Systems, which can Cause Chronic Constipation. Yes, his Flesh is CONSUMED AWAY, so that it cannot be Seen; and his Bones, which were not Seen, are now Sticking Out. Yes, his Body draws near to the Grave: because of Wasting Away, and his Spirit is Ready for the Angel of Death: beCause he is Fasting, having no Appetite to Eat nor Drink anything: beCause of his Terrible Sickness and Disease.

04-012 [_] However, if there is an Honest Messenger, or Good News Reporter among them — even one who Loves the Whole Truth about all Important Subjects, even an Interpreter of Dark

Sayings, being one Wise Man among a thousand Ignorant Fools — in Order to Show to the Sick Soul the Reason that Men were made to Walk UPRIGHTLY on 2 Feet — so that they might Pick Sweet Fruits from the Trees of Life, if they Repent and Return to the Garden of True Pleasures — then God is Gracious to him, and says: "Deliver him from going down into the Pit — I have found an Atonement for him." And thus such a Man is Healed when he Feasts on those Sweet Ripe Fresh Fruits from the Trees of Life. Yes, his Flesh shall become Fresher than the Flesh of a Child, and he shall Return to the Kind of a Person that he was during the Days of his Youth — he shall Pray to the Supreme Ruler for Forgiveness, and he will be Favorable to him, and have Mercy on him: beCause God always Favors his Obedient Children, even as any Good Father does; and therefore, he will See the Face of God with Great Joy when he Looks into the Mirror of Truths: beCause God will Give to the Humble man his own Righteousness in Holiness.

04-013 [_] Indeed, God Looks down on the Children of Unclean Men, and if any of them say: "I have Sinned, I have Broken your Laws, I have Disobeyed your Commandments, I have done Evil in your Sight, and Perverted that which was Right and Good, and it did not Profit me anything," then the Supreme Ruler will have Mercy on him and Deliver his Soul from going down into the Grave, into that Deep Dark Pit; and his Eyes will See the Light of Truths, which will Give to him Life when he Learns and Obeys those Great Truths.

04-014 [_] Behold, all of those Good Things the Supreme Ruler often Works with the Humble Honest Men, in Order to bring Back their Souls from the Pits of Self-destruction, in Order to be Enlightened with the Light of the Living God, who Created every Body to Heal itself, and to Regenerate itself by Means of Fasting and Praying, combined with certain Days of Feasting on Sweet Ripe Fresh Fruits from the Trees of Life. But, all of these Good Things are HIDDEN from the Proud People, who Look to their own misunderstandings, who put their Trust in the Vain wisdom of Unclean Men, who have Forsaken the Path of True Nolij, who have Wandered down Forbidden Paths of Self-destruction, and will not Confess all of their Sins, including all of their Dietary Sins, and how they have Polluted the Earth with their Abominations.

04-015 [_] Mark my Words of Truths, O Jobe — Listen to me with both of your Inner Ears, hold your Peace within you, and I will Speak with your Conscience. Moreover, if you have anything to Say, after my Speech is Finished, then Answer me: beCause I Seek to Justify you for your Righteousness. But, if you do not have an Answer, then Listen Intently to me — hold your Peace within you, and I will Teach to you True Wisdom and Profound Truths, which no Man can Prove to be WRong. — The New MAGNIFIED Version (NMV) of Jobe 33:14—33, in Plain English.

04-016 [_] And one of the Gods said, "Let us make Mankind in our own Image, according to our own Likeness, having Spirits, Minds, and Bodies like our own, whereby they can Choose for themselves what is Good for them to Eat and Drink: because of having the Freedom to do so, whereby they can Act Wisely, and thus become like us in all Ways, whereby they will Qualify to Govern their very own Worlds, even as we Govern them, which Worlds can be Created and Managed According to their Wills and Desires, whereby they can be Happy with themselves." — NMV of *Genesis 1:26*.

04-017 [_] And the God of this World said to those Spirits, "Behold, I have Given to you every Clean Green Herb that Bears Seeds, which is on the Surface of all of the Land on the Earth; and I

34

have also Given to you every Tree that Bears Sweet Fruits and Nuts, whose Seeds are within the Flesh of the Fruits — to you I have Given every Clean Green Herb and every Sweet Ripe Fruit and every Sweet Nut for Foods. Therefore, be Wise for yourselves, and Choose what is Good for you among all such Foods: because Satan has also Transplanted many Bad Fruits and Nuts and Herbs into this World of Woes from other Worlds of Lower Orders: because he Seeks to Rule Over you by Means of Deceptions and Lies, which Fruits and Herbs are Poisonous to Eat, which is why those Trees and Bushes are covered with Thorns, in Order to Warn you that they may Ruin your Precious Teeth, or even make you Sick, even though some of those Fruits are Good for making Juices, which are Good for Cleaning Out your Bowels, if you become Constipated by Eating Flesh of Beasts, Cheeses, Refined Sugars, Refined Grains, Eggs, and other Sticky Substances. After all, Satan is Testing your Spirits, whereby I may Discover who Loves me. Moreover, I have Given to every Beast of the Earth, and to every Fowl of the Air, and to every Creature that Creeps on the Earth, their own Special Diets, whereby you can Observe them, and thus Discover what is more Profitable for you to Eat. Yes, I have Given all such Things to every Creature, wherein there is the Spirit of Life, whereby they may Choose what is Good for them, even every Green Leaf and every Clean Herb, with the Seeds thereof for Foods: because every Creature must Eat. However, when they have Eaten too much, and have Lost their Appetites, they will Stop Eating, whereby they will Recover. Therefore, be Wise for yourselves, and do Likewise when you Lose your Appetites. In other Words, Eat when you are Hungry, and do not Eat when you are not Hungry; and Remember that Hunger is an Intense Appetite to Eat, and not the Time of Day, whereby you Form Bad Eating Habits." And so it was that when those Spirits were Born into Bodies on the Earth, they Instinctively Knew what to Eat. — NMV of *Genesis 1:29.*

04-018 [_] Of every Fruit Tree of the Garden of God, you may freely Eat According to your Appetites. — NMV of *Genesis 2:16.*

04-019 [_] And Jesus said to me, "Do not Seal the Sayings of the Prophecy of this little Book: because the Time is at Hand, and the Day of Judgment is soon to come, when he that is Unjust, shall still be Unjust; and he who is Filthy, shall still be Filthy; and he who is Righteous, shall still be Righteous; and he who is Holy, shall still be Holy: because the Grave has no Power to Transform Unclean People into Holy People. Behold, I come Quickly; and my Reward shall be with me — to Give to every Man According as his Works have been — and if his Works have been Evil: beCause of Believing the Lies of Satan, the Devil, he will be Given an Evil Reward in the Unholy Kingdom of Satan, the Devil; but, if his Works have been Good, he will be Given a Good Reward in the Holy Kingdom of All that is Good. Yes, I am the Alpha and the Omega, even the Beginning and the End of all Good Things — the First and the Last Man, himself, and the only Supreme Ruler of this Heaven and this Earth, which has been Committed to me by my Heavenly Father, since I have been Proven to be Worthy of it, having Passed all of the Tests of my Soul in other Worlds, whereby I Qualified to be the Supreme Ruler of this World, having Passed all of the Tests of my Soul from before the Foundation of this World, and having Passed all of the Tests of my Soul in this World, for which I have been Glorified by my Heavenly Father, who Sent me into this World to be your Anointed Savior and Righteous King.

04-020 [_] "Therefore, I have Taught to you my Father's Commandments, and Blest are they who Learn and Obey his Commandments: so that they might have a Right to Enter in through those Pearly White Gates, which Signify the Purity of the Mind, Spirit and Body of whomever is Entering into that Holy City, in Order to Feast on the Sweet Fruits from the Tree of Life: beCause, on the Outside of that Holy City, are the Filthy Hogs, Gluttons, Barking Dogs, Drunkards, Stinking Skunks, Poisonous Snakes, Drug Addicts, Filthy Sodomites, Prostitutes, Whoremongers, Warmongers, Murderers, Idolaters, and whosoever Loves and makes up Lies. Therefore, I, the Anointed Savior, have Sent to you my Angel to Testify to you about all of these Things, which should be Taught in all Churches, Worldwide.

04-021 [_] "Moreover, I am the Root from which King David Sprang, and I am his Offspring, also, being called the Father of Spirits, the Bright and Morning Star, the Holy One of the Household of Israel, the Wonderful Counselor, the Mighty God, the Prince of Peace, the Everlasting Father, the Redeemer of Mankind, the KING of Kings, and the RULER of Rulers. Therefore, the Holy Spirit and Bridegroom say: COME. Therefore, let the Bride also say: COME; and let him or her that is Thirsting for Truths, COME. Yes, whosoever is Willing to Repent, may come to the Fountain of Youth, in Order to Fill his or her Thirsty Soul with the Water of Life, which he or she may take Freely, and Drink until his or her Soul is Satisfied." — NMV of *Revelation 22:10—17*.

04-022 [_] And they said to me: What does the River of Water, which our Father saw, Mean? And I said to them that the Water that my Father saw was Symbolical of Filthiness; and his Mind was so Swallowed Up with other Thoughts, that he did not even Notice the Filthiness of the Water, which was Contaminated by the Industries of the Filthy People, who Produced Various Kinds of Abominations. And I said to them that it was an Awful Gulf, which Separated the Wicked Ones from the Tree of Life, and also from the Holy Ones of the Supreme Ruler, who would not Touch any such Abominations. And I said to them that it was a Representation of that Awful Hellish Condition, which the Angel said to me was Prepared for the Wicked Ones. And I said to them that our Father also saw that the Justice of the Supreme Ruler also Divided the Wicked Ones from the Righteous Ones; and the Brightness thereof was like the Brightness of a Flaming Fire, which ascends up to the Supreme Ruler forever and ever, and has no End: because he is the God of Justice.

04-023 [_] And they said to me, Does this thing mean the Torment of the Body during the Days of Probation, when Men are Tested during this Life; or, does it mean the Final State of the Spirit after the Death of the Temporal Body, or does it speak of the things which are Temporal, only? And it came to pass that I said to them that it was a Representation of things which are BOTH Temporal AND Spiritual: because the Day should come that they must be Judged according to their Works, yes, even the Works that were done by the Temporal Body during the Days of their Probation.

04-024 [_] Therefore, if they should Die in their State of Wickedness, they must be Cast Off, also, as to the Things that are pertaining to Righteousness; therefore, they must be brought to Stand in front of the Supreme Ruler, in Order to be Judged by their Works; and, if their Works have been Filthiness, they must needs be FILTHY; and, if they are Filthy, it must needs be that they cannot Dwell in the Kingdom of Holiness; if so, the Kingdom of God must be Filthy, also. But, behold, I say to you, the Kingdom of All that is Good is NOT Filthy, nor can any Unclean Thing Enter into that Holy Kingdom of Purity. Therefore, there must needs be a Place of

Filthiness, which is Prepared in Advance for that which is Filthy, which is Unclean, Rotten, Stinking, and Putrid. And there is just such a Place, which is already Prepared for the Devil and his Evil Followers; yes, it is that Awful Hellish Condition of which I have Spoken, and the Devil is the Founder of it: because he is the Enemy of All that is Good, which is God. Therefore, the Final State of the Souls of Men is to Dwell in the Holy Kingdom of All that is Good, or to be Cast Out of this World into a Lower Order of Worlds: beCause of that Justice of which I have Spoken, which Separates the Righteous Ones from the Wicked Ones. Therefore, the Wicked Ones are Rejected from the Righteous Ones, and also from that Tree of Life in the Paradise of Peace and True Happiness, whose Fruits are most Precious and most Desirable above all other Fruits; yes, it is the Greatest of all of the Gifts of the Gods: because a Person may Feast on those Good Fruits, and Live Forever in the House of Praise, in the Blest Land of Perfect Oneness, in the Paradise of Peace and True Happiness, where the little Birds of Cheerfulness are Singing, and the Fragrant Flowers are Blooming. And thus I Spoke to my Brothers, whose Spiritual Ears were Filled with the Wax of Unbelief, whereby they could not Hear what I was Saying with their Spiritual Ears, whereby they did not Understand me, and thus Deprived themselves of the Greater Things in Life. And so it is, Amen. — NMV of *First Nephi 15:26—36,* in Plain English.

04-025 [_] And now, my Sons, I would that you should Look to the Great Mediator between the Gods and Mankind, who is Jesus Christ; and Listen to his Great Commandments: because they are very Good for all of Mankind to Love and Obey, whereby they Liberate us from the Chains of Satan, and the Shackles of Sins; and be Faithful to his Inspired Words of Provable Truths, and Choose All that is Good, whereby you may have Eternal Life, according to the Will of his Holy Spirit, who would have all People to Repent; and not Choose Eternal Death, according to the Will of the Flesh and the Evils that are therein, which give the Devil Power to Captivate you, in Order to bring you Down into that Hellish Condition: so that he might Rule Over you in his own Evil Kingdom, which is Full of Filthy Greasy Things. — NMV of *Second Nephi 2:28—29.*

04-026 [_] And Jesus called a little Child to him, and set him in the midst of them, and said: "Truly I say to you, except you Humble yourself by Means of Fasting, until you are Converted, and thus become Like this little Child, having a Clean Body and a Pure Mind, you shall not Enter into the Holy Kingdom that is coming from Heaven to the Earth, which will be Established during the Last Days. Therefore, whomsoever shall Humble himself by Means of Fasting and Praying, until he is Converted in his Body and Mind, until he becomes Like this little Child, the same Person is Like the Greatest Person in the Kingdom of Heaven: because it is made up of Holy People, who are as Innocent as this little Child, who have Overcome the Devil with all of his Temptations, and are Free from the Prison of Sins. — See *Matthew 18 and the Book of Revelation.*

04-027 [_] Yes, come to him, and Offer your whole Soul — both Body, Mind and Spirit — as an Offering to him; and Continue with Fasting and Praying, and Endure unto the End of your Purification, even as all of the Holy Prophets Endured; and as the Supreme Ruler Lives, so shall you be Saved from all of your Sins, and thus be Reserved for a Position within that Holy Kingdom of All that is Good, which was Prepared for you from before the Foundation of this World. — NMV of *Omni 26.*

04-028 [_] Yes, he says: Come unto me, and you will Partake of the Sweet Fruits from the Tree of Life; yes, you shall Eat the Bread of Life, and Drink the Water of Life Freely, which is the Juice from those Sweet Fruits, as well as Coconut Water. — NMV. (See *Alma 5:34.*)

04-029 [_] He who has an Ear that can Hear, let him Hear what the Spirit says to the Churches of Confusion: To him who Overcomes all of his Sins, and gets the Victory over that Devil, I will Give to him the Fruits from the Tree of Life to Eat, and he will be Satisfied in the Midst of the Paradise of Peace and True Happiness. — NMV of *Revelation 2:7.*

04-030 [_] Because you have Patiently Kept my Words, and Obeyed my Commandments, I will also Keep you Safe from the Hour of Temptation, which will come on all of the Remainder of the People of the World, in Order to Test them who Dwell on the Earth, in Order to Try their Spirits, even as Metal Swords are Tested in the Furnace of Afflictions: so that they might be Proven to be Worthy for Battle during the Future. — NMV of *Revelation 3:10.*

04-031 [_] And to the Angel of the Church of the Laodicians, write: These Things says the Amen — the Faithful and True Witness, the Beginning of the Creation of the Most High Ruler of this Solar System — I Know your Works, that you are neither Hot nor Cold, neither For nor Against me. However, I Desire that you are either Hot or Cold: because I Hate the Luke-warmness of People. So then, beCause you are Lukewarm, and neither Hot nor Cold, I will Spit you Out of my Mouth, so to speak: because you say, "I am Rich, and increased with Goods, and have need of nothing" — and yet you do not Know that you are WRETCHED, MISERABLE, POOR, BLIND, and even NAKED! Therefore, I Counsel you to Buy Gold from me, which has been Tested in the Fire, even in the Furnace of Afflictions: so that you might be Truly Rich; and put on the White Clothing of Righteousness: so that you might be Clothed, and so that the Shame of your Nakedness does not Appear, as it now does; and Anoint your Eyes with Eye Salve: so that you might See the Meanings of the Words of Truths in their Brightness. Remember this — for as many People as I Love, I Rebuke and Chasten them for their Sins — be Zealous, therefore, and REPENT according to the Law of Repentance! Behold, I Stand at the Door of your Soul, and Knock on your Conscience, in Order to See if you are Alive, or Spiritually Dead. Therefore, if any Man Hears my Voice of Truths, and Opens the Door of his Heart, I will come into him, and will Feast with him, and he with me, you might say: because we will Communicate with each other both Day and Night. Therefore, to him who Overcomes all of his Sins, and Stops Sinning, I will Grant to him to Sit with me on my Throne of Glory — even as I also Overcame the Devil, and am now Sat Down with my Heavenly Father on his Great Throne. He who has an Open Ear, let him Hear what the Holy Spirit says to the Churches of Confusion. See *Revelation 3:14—22.*

04-032 [_] And Jesus lifted up his Eyes on his Self-disciplined Ones, and said: "Blest are you who are Poor, Humble, Submissive, and Obedient: because your Inheritance is in the Holy Kingdom of All that is Good; but, Woe to you who are Rich, Proud, Stubborn, and Disobedient: because your Inheritance is in the Unholy Kingdom of All that is Evil. Blest are you who Hunger now: because you will be Filled with the Oil of Joy; but, Woe to you who are Full of Foods now: because you are like Vessels that are Stuffed with Waste Matter, which have no Space for any Truths nor Wisdom; and therefore, during the Day of Judgment, you will be like Empty Vessels that cannot Hold any Oil of Joy. Blest are you when Evil Men shall Hate you without a Justified Cause, and when they will Separate you from their Company, and shall Reproach you with Evil

Names, and Cast you Out of their Churches for Speaking the Truth, and also tell Slanderous Lies about you, in Order to Try to give to you an Evil Name, for my Sake: because Great shall be your Reward in the Holy Kingdom of All that is Good. Yes, REJOICE during that Time, O Healthy Happy Children of the Great King, and LEAP for JOY — for behold, your Reward shall be Everlasting Good Health in the Holy Kingdom of the Gods: because, in like manner their Fathers did the same Evil Things to the Holy Prophets; but, three Woes to you who are Selfishly Rich: because you have already Received your Consolations. Yes, Woe to you who are Full of Filth, and Accumulations of Poisons: because you shall Hunger and Thirst for the Truths that can Set you Free; but, you will not Find them: because you are Blinded to those Truths by Fighting Against the Light of Truths, rather than Walking with the Light behind you. Therefore, Woe to you who Laugh now, who Mock these Inspired Words of Divine Truths: because you will Weep and Howl and Mourn, when you find yourselves in that Awful Hellish Condition, when the Devil has you Captivated with his Addictive Foods, Drinks, and Drugs. Moreover, Woe to you when all Men shall Speak Well of you: because so did their Fathers to the False Prophets, who said that all is Well in the Cursed Land of the Spiritual Cowards, and in the Homeland of the Tax Slaves, Usury Slaves, Insurance Slaves, Drug Slaves, and Work Slaves. — NMV. (See *Luke 6:20—26.*)

04-033 [_] And Jesus Spoke a Parable to them, saying: Can the Blind People Properly Lead the Blind People? — will they not both Stumble and Fall into the Ditch, Together? He who says, "I See," is Surely the Most Blind: beCause of Assuming that he Sees All Things, when he does not See even one-hundredth of all that he Needs to See. Likewise, he who says, "I Hear," is Surely the Most Deaf, if he does not Realize that there are Mountains of Information that he has not yet Discovered, and especially if he cannot See nor Hear my Words of Truths, and Agree that he would do Well to be one of my Most Humble Disciples, who does not Presume anything. Indeed, the Disciple is not Above his Master; but, every Disciple shall do Well to be Perfected as his Master was Perfected. And why do you behold the Speck, which is in your Brother's Eye; but, Fail to See the Beam of Darkness in your own Eye? And how can you Rightly say to your Brother: "Brother, let me Pull Out the Speck that is in your Eye," when you yourself cannot See the Beam of Darkness in your own Eye: because it is Blinding you? O you Hypocrite, Cast the Beam Out of your own Eye, FIRST; and then you will See Clearly HOW to Pull the Speck Out of your Brother's Eye. Truly I say to you, if you were Holy, you would bring forth Holy Children; but, because you are Unclean, you bring forth Unclean Children, which is the Fruit of your Womb, even as a Healthy Tree brings forth Healthy Fruits; but, a Sick Tree brings forth Sick Fruits: beCause a Good Tree cannot bring forth Corrupt Fruits; neither does a Corrupt Tree bring forth Good Fruits. Indeed, every Tree is Known by its Fruits: because Men do not Gather Figs from Thorn Bushes, nor Grapes from Saw Vines, nor Dates from Cactus Plants. Therefore, a Good Man brings forth that which is Good from the Good Treasure Chest of his Bowels and Mind; and an Evil Man brings forth that which is Evil from the Evil Treasure Chest of his Bowels and Mind: beCause, out of the Abundance of whatever is in the Bowels and Mind, the Mouth Speaks. And why do you call me your Lord and Master, saying: "Lord, Lord," but Refuse to Do the Good Things that I Teach to you? — NMV of *Luke 6:39—46.*

04-034 [_] Then his Mother and his Brothers came to him, and could not come near to him because of the Multitude of People. And the News was passed on from one to another, until it was told to him by certain People, who said: "Your Mother and Brothers stand Outside, desiring to See you." And Jesus Answered them: "My Mother and my Brothers are these People who Hear the Words of the Supreme Ruler, and Obey them." — NMV of *Luke 8:19—21.*

04-035 [_] Whosoever therefore shall be Ashamed of me and of my Lovable Words of Provable Truths during this Adulterous and Sinful Generation, of him will the Son of the Man of Holiness also be Ashamed when he comes with the Glory of his Holy Father in a Great Spaceship, and with the Multitude of his Holy Angels in their Flying Saucers, in Order to Gather Out his Elected Servants from the far ends of the Earth, in Order to Determine who is Worthy to Rule with me over all of the Nations of the World in that Holy Kingdom, which will be Established over all Nations during the Last Days, after the Spirits of Mankind have been Tested." — NMV of *Mark 8:38.*

04-036 [_] And when Jesus came to his Disciples, he saw a great Multitude of People around them, and the Scribes were Questioning them. And when the People saw the Face of Jesus, they were Greatly Amazed, and ran up to him and Saluted him. And he asked the Scribes: "What are you Questioning among yourselves?" And one of the Multitude Answered, "Master, I have brought to you my Son, which has an Unclean Spirit in him, and it makes him Dumb: so that he cannot Speak; and wherever that Spirit takes him, he Claws at himself, and he Foams at his Mouth, and Gnashes with his Teeth, and Pines away; and I spoke to your Disciples, saying that they could Cast him Out; but, they could not do it. Therefore, can you Help him?" And Jesus Answered, "O Faithless Generation, how long shall I be with you? How long shall I Allow you to go on in your State of Ignorance? Bring him to me."

04-037 [_] And they brought him to Jesus; and when he saw Jesus, the Evil Spirit immediately caused him to Tear his Clothing, and to Claw himself with his Fingernails; and he Fell Naked to the Ground, and Wallowed in the Dirt, while Foaming at his Mouth. And Jesus Asked his Physical Father: "How long ago was it since this Evil Spirit came into him?" And he said, "Since he was a Child. Moreover, it has often Cast him into the Fire, and into the Water, in Order to Try to Destroy him; but, if you can do anything to Save him, please have Compassion on us, and Help us: because we Believe in you, and Trust you to do Good for us, even though we are not Worthy of your Blessings."

04-038 [_] Jesus said to him, "If you can Believe it, all Good Things are Possible to him who Believes." And straightway the Father of the Child Cried Out, and said with Tears: "Master, I Believe — please Help my Unbelief." Therefore, when Jesus saw that the People came running Together, he Rebuked the Evil Spirit, saying to him: "You Deaf and Dumb Spirit, I Charge you to come Out of him, and do not Enter into him again."

04-039 [_] And thus the Evil Spirit caused the Man to Cry, and Tore at his Soul, as if to Kill him; but, it still came Out of him; and he that was Possessed by that Evil Spirit was like a Dead Man, insomuch that many People said, "He is DEAD!" But, Jesus took him by the Hand, and Lifted him Up; and thus he arose and stood on his Feet. And when Jesus came into the House where he was staying, his Disciples Asked him privately: "Why could we not Cast him Out?" And he said to them, "This Kind of an Unclean Spirit can only be Cast Out by Fasting and Praying." — NMV of *Mark 9:14—29.*

04-040 [_] So, the People of Nineveh Believed what was Revealed about the Supreme Ruler, and Proclaimed a Fast, and put on Sackcloth, from the Greatest of them to the Least of them: because the Words of Truths that Jonah had Taught to them came to the King of Nineveh, and he arose from his Throne, and laid aside his Robe from him, and covered himself with Sackcloth, and sat in Ashes. Moreover, he caused it to be Proclaimed and Published throughout all of Nineveh, by the Decree of the King and his Nobles, saying: "Let neither Man nor Beast, Herd nor Flock, Taste of anything; let them not Eat, nor Drink Water; but, let both Men and Beasts be covered with Sackcloth, and Cry Mightily to the God of Jonah; yes, let them Turn everyone away from his Evil Ways, and from the Violence that is Worked by Hands: because who can tell if God will Turn Away his Wrath, and Relent; and Turn Away his Fierce Anger, so that we do not Perish? Therefore, let everyone Fast and Pray for the next 40 Days and 40 Nights, while we Patiently Wait on our Creator God, with Weeping and with Mourning for all of the Sins that we have Committed against him in our State of Ignorance. Let us do as Jonah has said, and use Water to Flush Out our Bowels every Day, until the Water comes Out as Clear as Water; and let us take Daily Baths in Water, after we have sat in the Ashes, Begging for Mercy and Pardon, being covered with Sackcloth and the Shame of our Uncleanness.

04-041 [_] And God saw their Works, that they Ceased from them, and Turned from their Evil Ways; and thus the Supreme Ruler Relented of the Evil that he had said that he would Do to them, and he did not Do it: because they Repented according to the Law of Repentance. — NMV of *Jonah 3:5—10.*

04-042 [_] Truly I say to you, that during the Day of Judgment, the Men of Nineveh shall rise up and Condemn this Generation of Evildoers: because they Repented according to the Preaching of Jonah; and behold, a Greater Prophet than Jonah is now here. (See *Matthew 12:41.*)

04-043 [_] Then Jesus was Led by the Spirit of God into the Wilderness, in Order to be Tempted by the Devil, in Order to Prove that he could Overcome him. And when Jesus had Fasted for 40 Days and 40 Nights, without Eating, he was very Hungry. And when the Tempter came to him, he said: "If you are the Son of God, then Command that these Stones are made into Foods." But, Jesus Answered him, "It is Written that Mankind shall not Live by Foods alone; but, by Means of every Word that proceeds out of the Mouth of the Supreme Ruler." {FOOTNOTE: EVERY Word would include the *Old Testament,* and especially in the Light of the Fact that the *Old Testament* was the ONLY Existing Scriptures during that Time, when Jesus said those Inspired Words! Selah. Selah means to STOP and THINK. Therefore, STOP and Think about that common Phrase, which some Foolish People make, who say: "We do not Live by the OLD Testament; but, we Live by the NEW Testament, only" Therefore, such Foolish People never read all of those Scriptures that I have Quoted, which Relate with Fasting; and therefore, they are Blinded to all of that Great Truth. Indeed, those Lazy People are some of the most Ignorant, Proud, and Insane Idiots that you will ever Meet: because they Deprive themselves of such Enlightening Books as *Deuteronomy, Isaiah, Jeremiah, Ezekiel, Amos, Proverbs, Pslams, Job, Daniel,* and so on. In Fact, they Deprive themselves of LIFE, itself, and end up in some Sanitized Slaughterhouse, getting their Precious Million-dollar Organs removed with 10-cent Razor Blades, you might say! Therefore, be Wise for yourself, and do not be LAZY; but, Study all of the *Scriptures* that you can Find, which includes any and all of my Sacred Writings: because they are also Inspired by the Great Creator God, who has been Teaching New Lessons to me for 50+

Years, which everyone will do Well to Learn: so that they do not have to Repeat the very same Mistakes that I have made, just to Learn those same Good Lessons. Indeed, that is the very Reason that I have taken so much Time to Write all of these Important Things — not because I need the Exercise, only; but, that you Need to Learn what I have Learned. Moreover, we all Need to Learn from our Mistakes, no matter who Reveals them; but, we do not Need to Waste our Precious Time reading Trash Literature, such as Romance Novels and Comic Books: beCause Life is just too Short. Neither do we Need to Waste our Time Watching Worthless Television Programs, if there is nothing Educational to Watch, such as those Commercial Advertisements, which use up one-third of our Time, even while Watching News Reports. Indeed, suppose that I stopped giving to you Quotes from the *Scriptures,* about every other Page, and Wasted your Time with Advertisements for Coffee, Cokes, and Hamburgers — would you be bothered to read this Book? Of course not! So, why be bothered to Watch such Advertisements on TV? Why not Live within a Swanky Fortress, which has nothing but Honest News Reports and Truly Educational Programs to Watch, having all of that other Trash Screened Out: beCause it is not Necessary for Living a Good Life? End of Note.}

04-044 [_] Then the Devil took him up into the Holy City, and set him on a Pinnacle of the Temple, and said to him: "If you are the Son of God, then cast yourself down: because it is written, He shall give his Angels Charge concerning you; and in their Hands they will bear you up, lest at any Time you dash your Foot against a Stone and Fall." And Jesus said to him, "It is written again, You shall not Tempt the Creator, your Supreme Ruler." {NOTE: Tens of thousands of Foolish People TEMPT the Creator by doing such Insane Things as High-wire Walking, Racing Cars, Jumping Motorcycles across Cars and even Canyons, and Playing all Kinds of Dangerous Games, which are called SPORTS; but, notice how EASY it is to get Hurt, and then Suffer for Days, Weeks, Months, Years, and sometimes for Life — just for PRIDE and Foolishness. (Remember Christopher Reeves of Superman Fame, who was only able to Wiggle his Fingers after Years of Paralysis from falling off of a Horse while Playing his Favorite Sport.) Therefore, I can tell you plainly that any Kind of Competition is a SIN: beCause it is Impossible to Compete without Anxiety, Stress, Fear, Worry, Tension, Pride, and the Diseases that accompany such People as those who make a Career out of it. (Think of Mohammed Ali, the Famous Boxer, for a Good Example of one who went to the Extremes, who was Humiliated until his Death with a Defective Brain.) Therefore, if you Want to Avoid such Humiliations, just Humble yourself and GIVE UP all such Competition: because you can Live a much Healthier and Happier Life without it. Indeed, anything that Causes you to get Upset, or Afraid, is WRONG, and can do much Damage to your Nervous System. Therefore, do not give a Speech, nor get into any Argument, if it is Upsetting to you: because it is a Sin to you. Just keep SILENT, and hold your Peace within you: because it is not Worth the Price you will Pay for it. For Example, if you attend some Meeting, such as a Church Gathering, and you Know that those People do not Agree with the Truths that you Believe, be Wise, and only Ask Questions, as if you were a little Child: because, if you cannot get those People to THINK, you cannot Teach anything to them: because their Minds are already set on whatever they Believe, even if their Beliefs are False. Therefore, you have to make a Way for yourself in Order to Teach something to them, by Asking them Questions that they cannot Answer, which Causes them to Ask you for the Answer, at which Time you can Teach the Truth to them with LOVE, as if they were Ignorant and Innocent little Children. In other Words, do not Expect them to Know all that you Know; but, be very Patient with them: because they have much to Learn. However, in this Fast-paced Society, there is not Enough Time to hold Rational Conversations with other People, like it was a thousand Years ago: because they are already Late for the next Appointment, or whatever. Therefore, you might Accomplish much more, if you simply offer to them a Copy of this Book, and say: "I think that you would do Well to read this Book with an Open Mind, and do not Presume that you already Know what it Reveals: because you do not Know, if you have not Studied it." Moreover, while you are saying it, you must Look straight into their Eyes, and say it with Sternness; but, also with the Spirit of Love: because Love is what other People like most, and after that they like the Whole Truth, even if it Proves their Beliefs to be WRong: because they Sense that only the Truth can Liberate them from the Prison of Lies. Therefore, if you are a Good Example of someone who has Cleaned House by Fasting and Praying, they will be Converted to that Truth, or else they will go straight to Hell for Rejecting it; but, only if you are a Holy Person: because a Bad Example can be Worse than no Example at all, which explains WHY that I do not put my own Picture on this Inspired Book: because I am NOT a Good Example of a Holy Man; but, I Know what such a Man Looks like, and I also Know that I have Looked the same Way during Times past: because I Dedicated myself to that Cause; but, as I have Explained elsewhere, I could not Maintain that Higher State of Good Health: beCause of being all alone among Professing "Christians," who had no Interest in Holiness of Mind, Spirit, and Body, and certainly no Interest in Supporting someone who could Prove them to be Wrong concerning almost all Doctrines, which Truths they Rejected and "went to Hell," as they say; but, they also Managed to Drag me down with them to some Degree: because they Refused to Strengthen me in my Quest to do what was and still is RIIT. Therefore, I have resorted to an Effort to Enlighten such People's Minds with Inspired Words of Provable Truths, with the Hope that they might some Day Realize their Grave Mistake, and REPENT; and then be more Willing to Help others to Repent, rather than Deny all of this Great Truth, and end up in that Sanitized Slaughterhouse, which, by the Grace of God, I will Avoid: because God has Mercy on those People who have Mercy on others; and I have shown as much Mercy and Compassion as anyone on this Earth, as far as I Know, when it comes to telling the Truth: because I have Sincerely told all of the Truths that have come to my Mind, which everyone should Accept, unless they can Prove those Truths to be WRong — either by becoming Holy, and Maintaining that Holiness, or else Prove it to be WRong by Reason and Logic. However, most People are not the slightest bit Interested in Proving anything: because they are Brainwashed with Lies, and quite Contented to go to Hell, while saying that they are going to Heaven; but, only the Holy Ones will have any Part in the Government of God, which most certainly EXCLUDES them: because they Deny the entire Doctrine of Holiness, and say that we are all Saved by Grace, alone, which is the Truth; but, they Misunderstand how Grace Works. Yes, they Forget that Song that says: "There, but for the Grace of God, go I." In other Words, we could have been Born in another Bodies in other Places, and would have never Learned what we have now Learned. For Example, you are just one of the very FEW People who are Reading this very Book, or Listening to it, by the Grace of God: because you could have been Blinded to it by your Pride; but, because of being Humble, you are now Reading it, or Listening to it, even if you are Humble because of being Humiliated by some Sickness or Disease or Accident, which has Caused you to Want to Learn more about Fasting. Therefore, we get "Grace for Grace," as it states in *John 1:16.* In other Words, when we show others Mercy and Grace, we get more Mercy and Grace; but, when we have the Spirit of Greed and Selfishness, and only seek to take Advantage of others, we are certainly NOT going to get the Grace of God to Overcome our Sins. Moreover, we are on this Sinking Ship Together, whether we like it or not; and therefore, we must Seek each others Salvation, even if we all have to make some Sacrifices, and go Sell all that we have: so that we might Band Together, in Order to Build a New Jerusalem: beCause it is our only Hope for Physical Salvation, which will also get Done by GRACE: because it will Require the Grace of God to Change the Minds of so many People, who have been Humiliated for so long; but, they are still PROUD and FOOLISH, thinking that they can be Independent Jackasses, and also be Saved. [See www.Amazon.com for: **"The Loathsome Burdens of the Independent Jackasses!" (A New Approach for Solving our Massive Problems!) By The Worldwide People's Revolution!® Book 051.**] Yes, they Conveniently Forget that we are all Members of each other — no matter how Weak and Sinful we are — and therefore, the Weaker we are, the more we Need the Help of others to Overcome our Weaknesses. (See *Romans 12.*) Indeed, it would be Wonderful if all People in the entire World could See the Vision of Holiness, and then make WAR on Filthiness, Pollution, Crimes, Poverty, and WAR, itself, by Building those **"GLORIOUS Swanky Hotels Castles and Fortresses!" (Beautiful Planned City States for WISE Intelligent Well-Educated People with Common Sense and Good Understanding!),** which would Solve at least 248 Massive Problems, Worldwide, including Pollution, Waste Disposal, Crimes, Poverty, and WARS; but, instead, only a very FEW People can See the Vision, and they are all somewhat like Helpless Chickens, Peahens, Sheeps, and Goats, you might say, who can only make NOISES among ROARING Lions, HOWLING Wolves, BARKING Dogs, GROWLING Bears, Sneaky Snakes, Stinking Skunks, and a Host of Filthy Cockroaches, Fleas, and Spiders, which Poisonous Spiders Weave very Complicated Webs, which not only Trap themselves; but, they Trap everyone who comes near to them: because of the Deceptions of Capitalism, Competition, and FOOLISHNESS that is all DOOMED with the Devil who Inspired it. [See: **"The Nature of CAPITALISM!" (A List of the EVILS of CAPITALISM!) By The Worldwide People's Revolution!® Book 038.**] In Fact, while Professing "Christians" are Competing for Gain, they are all going to Hell, Together, rather than Band Together with a Common Cause, in Order to Save themselves from their Sins, Sicknesses, Diseases, Plagues, Wars, and Deaths — all of which is the Result of Rejecting TRUTHS without any Just Causes, such as the Truth about the Need for a Holy City, which does not Allow Unclean People to Enter into that most Holy Court, which is the Innermost Court, which gives to everyone an Incentive for Striving to get there: because it contains those **"Beautiful Swanky PALACES"** for Holy People. Therefore, will you Help me to Build it, or will you go to Hell with all of the other Unbelievers, who Reject that Great Truth, while Trying in Vain to SURVIVE among the People who are like Lions and Wolves? What will it Require for People to Understand that without **"The New RIGHTEOUS One-World Government,"** there is NO Hope? And, in Order to Establish that Good Government, you must Help me to SPREAD this Message, by SHARING my Good Books with others: so that they might See the Vision of a Holy City, and at last VOTE for it: beCause THAT is how Dumbmocracy Works. Otherwise, we will all end up in the Valley of Armageddon, getting a Bloodbath, in Order to Cleanse our Minds of such Foolishness as Competition, so-called "Independence," and PRIDE, which comes before Destruction. End of Note.}

04-45 [_] Again, the Devil took him up into an exceeding High Mountain, and showed to him all of the Kingdoms of the World with a Big Telescope, and the Glory of each of them; and said to him: "I will Give to you all of these Things, if you will fall down and Worship me." Then Jesus said to him, "Get yourself Away from here, Satan: because it is written, 'You shall Worship the Creator, your Supreme Ruler, and him only shall you Serve.' And that is what I am going to Do." Then the Devil left him there to Freeze; but, behold, Holy Angels came and Ministered to him.

(See *Matthew 4:1—11.*) {NOTE: There are NO Angels Ministering to anyone, Today, as far as I Know, even though it Appears more Necessary now than ever; but, because there is no Holy Church, nor even a Congregation of Righteous People, there is no Good Reason for Angels to Appear: because it Requires at least 2 to 3,000 Humble People, who are Gathered Together in his Name, just to Build a Holy City, whereby everyone can have Good Foods to Eat; but, what about Clean Air to Breathe, and Living Water to Drink? Yes, what about Acid Rains and POLLUTION all around the World, which Blows in the Wind all over the World? Stand UP, O Righteous Man, and tell me WHERE a Body can Live in this Insane World as a Holy Man? And how long can he Live there, before the Pollution, Crimes, and Wars are at his own Doorsteps? Therefore, we MUST take Over this Insane World, at whatever the Cost, and Straighten it out with **"The Swanky Sword of Divine Truths!"** because, if Truths cannot Straighten it out, nothing else can. Therefore, us your own Sword of Truths Wisely, while there is still some Air left to Breathe; and do not set your Heart on those "Vain Things of the World," which the Devil Tempts you to Lust after: because they will all Perish. End of Note.}

04-046 [_] And Moses said, "When I was gone up onto the Mount, in Order to Receive the Tablets of Stone, even the Tablets of the Covenant that the Creator made with you, then I stayed on the Mount for 40 Days and 40 Nights — I did not Eat Food nor Drink Water … And I fell down in front of the Creator, as at the first Time, for 40 Days and 40 Long Nights — I did not Eat Food, nor Drink Water; but, I Washed myself with Water, and Flushed Out my Bowels with Water every Day, by using a Gourd, which Joshua put up to my Hinder Parts full of Water, pouring it into my Bowels, even as you must also do for one another, in Order to be Saved from your Internal Filthiness, which is an Accumulation from Head to Toe of Uneliminated Waste Matter: because of Eating too much, or because of Eating Foods that are Unnatural for People to Eat: because the Perfect Food for Mankind is the Fresh Raw Sweet Fruits from the Tree of Life, plus some Clean Green Leaves, and a few Raw Nuts, as it was in the Beginning for Adam and Eve in the Garden of Eden." — NMV of Deuteronomy 9:9, and Verse 18.

04-047 [_] And Ahab told Jezebel all that Elijah had done, and how he had Slain all of the Unholy Prophets of Baal with the Sword. Then Jezebel sent a Messenger to Elijah, saying: "So let the Gods do to me, and more also, if I do not make your Life as the Life of one of those Prophets that you have Slain, by about this same Time, Tomorrow." And when Elijah saw the Message, he arose and went away for the Sake of his Life, and came to Beersheba, which belongs to Judah, and left his Servant there to Attend to his Garden.

04-048 [_] And Elijah went for a Day's Journey into the Wilderness, and came and sat down under a Juniper Tree, to get Out of the Hot Sunlight; and he Requested that he might Die, and said: "It is now Enough, O Creator; therefore, take away my Life: because I am no Better than my Fathers, who were all Sinners." However, as he lay by a little Campfire, during the Cool Night, and Slept under the Juniper Tree, behold, the Angel of the Creator Touched him on the Ribs, and said to him: "Arise, and EAT."

04-049 [_] And Elijah Looked, and behold, there was a Cake baked on the Coals of the Fire, being Wrapped up in Banana Leaves; and a Cruse of Water was at his Head. And he did Eat and Drank, and laid himself down again, and went to Sleep. And then the Angel of the Creator came again the second Time, and Touched him on the other Side of his Ribs, and said: "Arise, O

Elijah, and EAT: because the Journey is too long without a Full Stomach." And thus he Arose, and did Eat and Drank again, and then he went by the Strength of that Nourishment, which he got from Eating that Food, unto Mount Horeb, even to the Holy Mountain of the Supreme Ruler, where he Fasted for 40 Days and 40 Nights in a Cave, which also had a Stream of Water running through it, which he used to Flush Out his Bowels by Means of Enemas, and to take Daily Baths in that Water: because, like everything that we Clean, the Human Body is also Cleansed with Water, both Internally and Externally, even if that Water comes from Fruit and Vegetable Juices, without which we would all Die from Constipation: beCause we cannot Live Long without the Water of Life, much less Obtain Perfect Health by being Perfectly Cleansed from all Internal Filth, which can Reside within the Human Body for 40 Years or more. — NMV of *First Kings 19:1—8.*

04-050 [_] "… And that is not all. Do you not suppose that I Know of these Things, myself? Behold, I Testify to you that I do Know that these Things whereof I have Spoken are True. And how do you suppose that I Know of their Surety? Behold, I say to you that they are made Known or Revealed unto me by the Holy Spirit of the Supreme Ruler. Behold, I have Fasted and Prayed for many Days and long Nights: so that I might Learn these Things for myself. And now, I do Know for myself that they are True: beCause the Creator and Supreme Ruler has made them Known to me by his Holy Spirit …" — Alma 5:45—46.

04-051 [_] And the Lord God took the Man, and put him into the Garden of Eden, in Order to Dress the Trees, to Prune Out any Dead or Unwanted Limbs, and to Keep the Garden Neat. And thus the Ruling God Commanded the Man, saying: "Of every Fruit Tree of this Garden, you are Free to Eat; but, of the Fruit from the Tree of the Nolij of All that is Good and Evil, you shall not Eat it: because, during the Day that you Eat thereof, you shall Surely Die a Spiritual Death." — NMV of *Genesis 2:15—17.* See also *Second Peter 3:8, KJV.*

04-052 [_] This is the Punishment that a Man receives for Obeying the Voice of his Wife, when it is Contrary to the Laws of the Supreme Ruler — and to Adam he said: "Because you have Listened to the Voice of your Wife, and have Eaten from the Tree of which I Commanded you, saying: 'You shall NOT Eat from it' — Cursed is the Ground for your Sake — in Sorrow shall you Eat from it for all of the Remaining Days of your Life: because all Kinds of Varmints will Consume it, or Destroy it. Moreover, Thorns also and Thistles shall it bring forth to you; and you will Eat the Herbs of the Field, even the Seeds that are made for Birds and Cattle to Eat; yes, by the Sweat of your Face you shall Eat Foods, until you Return unto the Ground, yourself: because Out of the Ground you were taken, even from the Elements of the Dust: because Dust is what you are made of, and unto Dust you shall Return, which is True of all Creatures both Great and Small." (See *The NMV of Genesis 3:17—19.*)

04-053 [_] "And Enoch Walked with the Supreme Ruler; and the Supreme Ruler took him away to a Place called Mount Zion." (See *Genesis 5:24; Hebrews 11:5; and the Book of Moses &:69.*)

04-054 [_] Now the Creator had said to Abram, "Get you Out of your own Country, and Away from your Relatives, and Away from your Father's Household, unto a Land that I will Show to you, even a Land that is Choice above all other Lands; and I will make of you a Great Multitude of Nations, and I will Bless you, and make your Name very Great among all of the Nations:

because you have Loved me, and have Kept my Commandments; and therefore, you shall be a Blessing and a Cursing unto all Peoples: beCause of your Offsprings, who shall be both Good and Evil: because of being more Intelligent People, who will Use their Talents for both Good and Evil, whereby I will Test the Spirits of all Peoples. Indeed, I will Bless those People who Bless you, and Curse those who Curse you; and in you shall all of the Families of the Earth be Blest and Cursed: because of your Children, one of whom will be their Anointed Savior, who will Save all Souls who Believe in him and Love and Obey him: because he is their Great King, even from the Beginning, whose Spirit was Chosen from before the Foundation of this World to be the Father and Savior of it: because his Father found him Worthy in another World of a Higher Order." — NMV of *Genesis 12:1—3.*

04-055 [_] "Blest are the Meek, Teachable People: because they shall Inherit the Earth, not Heaven." (See *Matthew 5:5.*)

04-056 [_] "But the True Fast is this: Do nothing Wickedly during your Life; but, Serve the Supreme Ruler with a Pure Mind, and Keep his Commandments, and Live According to his Precepts; nor Allow any Wicked Desire to Enter into your Mind; but, Trust in the Creator, that if you do those Things, and Fear him, and ABSTAIN from EVERY EVIL WORK and FILTHY WORD, you shall Live unto God. Indeed, if you shall Do that, you shall Perfect a Great Fast, and an Acceptable one unto the Creator … This Fast, says he, while you do also Observe the Commandments of the Creator, is Exceedingly Good. Thus shall you therefore Keep it. First of all, take Heed to yourself, and Keep yourself from every Wicked Act, and from every Filthy Word, and from every Hurtful Desire; and Purify your Mind from all of the Vanity and Foolishness of this present World. Therefore, if you shall Observe those Things, this Fast shall be Right, and thus you shall be Justly Rewarded for it." (See *Similitude 5:5—7, and Verses 28—29,* in *the Lost Books of the Bible.*)

04-057 [_] "But they who are LAZY and SLOW TO PRAY, Doubt to Seek anything from the Great Creator God …"

A-[_] "For every Pure Body shall Receive its Reward, which is found without Spots, in which the Holy Spirit has been Appointed to Dwell …"

B-[_] "… Listen further, says he: Keep this Body of yours Clean and Pure, so that the Spirit that shall Dwell in it may bear Witness to it, and be Judged to have been with you. Also take Heed that it is not Instilled into your Mind that this Body Perishes, and that you therefore Abuse your Body for any Lust. For if you shall Defile your Body, you shall also at the same Time Defile the Holy Spirit; and if you shall Defile the Holy Spirit, you shall not Live in the Blest Land of Perfect Oneness with God." — NMV

C-[_] "… But now you must Guard yourself; and seeing that God is Almighty and Merciful, he will Grant a Remedy to what you have formerly done Amiss, if for the Time to come you shall not Defile your Body nor Spirit: because they are Companions Together, and the one cannot be Defiled without the other one being Defiled, also. Therefore, Keep both your Body and Mind PURE, and you shall Live unto God." — Similitude 5:39, 57, 58—59, and 62—63.

04-058 [_] "These Commands are Profitable to those Humble People who shall Repent of those Sins that they have formerly Committed — if for the Time to come they shall not continue in those same Sins. — Similitude 6:4.

04-059 [_] "He that gives himself up for just One Day to his Pleasures and Delights, and Does whatever Evil Thing his Soul Desires, if Full of Great Folly; nor does he Understand what he has Done; and the Day following he Forgets what he Did the Day before ..." — Similitude 6:35.

04-060 [_] "... You See therefore how that the Time of Worldly Enjoyments is but Short — but that of Pain and Torment is a great deal Longer." — Similitude 6:32.

04-061 [_] "... That is a Vain Pleasure to every Man which he does Willingly for an Evil Purpose." — Similitude 6:39.

04-062 [_] "... For by Forbearance and Humility of Mind, Men shall Attain unto Life, which Begins with Good Health; but, by Sedition and Contempt for the Laws of God, they shall purchase Sicknesses, Diseases, and Deaths unto themselves." — NMV of Similitude 8:64.

04-063 [_] "Do not seem to Consider — as if you were Wise — what you do not Understand; but, Pray to the Creator, your Supreme Ruler, that you may be Given the Ability to Understand it ..."

04-064 [_] "... Be not therefore Disquieted at those Things which you cannot See Clearly; but, get the Understanding of those Things which you can See Clearing. Forbear to be Curious, and I will Show to you all Things that I ought to Declare to you ..."

04-065 [_] "... So shall a Man Bear his Name in Vain, unless he shall also be Anointed with his Powers."

04-066 [_] "... For all of these Things I gave Thanks to the Creator, that being moved with Mercy towards all of those People upon whom his Name is called, he sent to us the Angel of Repentance, in Order to Preside over us who have Sinned against him; and that he has Refreshed our Spirits, which were almost gone, and who had no Hope of Salvation; but, we are now Refreshed by the Regeneration of Life."

04-067 [_] "So, when the Church of God shall be Purified — by the Wicked Ones and the Counterfeits being Cast Out; yes, by the Mischievous and the Doubtful, and all that have behaved themselves Wickedly in the World, and Committed Various Kinds of Sins, being Cast OUT — the True Church shall be of One Hope, One Understanding, One Opinion, One Faith, and of the same Charity." — Similitude 9:19, 20—21, 122, 135, 175.

04-068 [_] "No Man can Serve 2 Masters: because he will either Hate the one, and Love the other; or else he will Hold to the one, and Despise the other. Therefore, you cannot Serve both God and Materialism: because it brings in Confusion: because they are Contrary to one another. Likewise, if you Allow your Worldly Ambitions to Override your Spiritual Goals, you will Fail to Obtain those Goals: because it Requires a Total Commitment to one or to the other. Therefore, let him who puts his Hands to the Plow in the Field of Life, not Look Back with any Longing Desires for those Vain Things that cannot Satisfy the Soul; but, let him Look Straight Forward, and Persist toward his Goal unto the End of his Life." — NMV of *Matthew 6:24*.

04-069 [_] "Now, they who are Engaged in much Business, and in Diversities of Affairs, do not Join themselves to the Servants of God; but, they Wander Astray — being called away by those Affairs by Means of which their Spiritual Lives are CHOKED OUT."

04-070 [_] "Our Supreme Ruler and Creator, who Rules over all Good Things, and has Power over all of his Good Creatures, will not Remember our Offenses; but, he is easily Appeased by those Humble People who Confess their Sins, and Aknolij the Fact that Satan Rules over this World, and is the Master of all Evil People and Evil Creatures; but, a Proud Man, being Languid, Mortal, Infirm, and Full of Sins, Perseveres in his Anger against other Men — as if it were in his Power to Save or Destroy them." — NMV

04-071 [_] "But this present World, and all of the Vanities of their False Riches, must be Cut Off from them; and then they will be Fit for Services in the Kingdom of our God." — NMV

04-072 [_] "… And I say to you who have Received this Seal: Keep Simplicity and Humility, and do not Remember the Offenses which are Committed against you, nor continue in Malice, nor in Bitterness, through the Memory of Offenses."

04-073 [_] "… The Spirit of the Creator Dwells in those People who Love Peace: beCause Peace is Beloved; but, he is Far Off from the Contentious and Bitter People, and from those who are Full of Malice, which is an Intent to Injure someone." — NMV of Similitude 9:188, 208, 261, 264, and 269.

04-074 [_] "For if you Keep those Commands, all of the Lusts and Pleasures of this present Evil World shall be Subject to your Will; and Success shall Follow you in every Good Undertaking; but, only if you are Located in the Right Place, where there is more Traffic, and more Opportunities to Sell Things that you make with Hands, or Grow in your Garden." — NMV

04-075 [_] "… And they who do not Follow his Commands, shall Deliver themselves unto Sicknesses, Diseases, and Deaths of Various Kinds; and everyone who Engages in Wars shall be Guilty of his own Blood, as well as the Blood of any Innocent Souls whom he might Slay."

04-076 [_] "For he who Wants and Allows INCONVENIENCES in his Daily Life, is in Great Torment and Necessity: being Destitute of the Simplicity of the Kingdom of our God, whereby each Soul does only one Thing at a Time, and does it very Well, being Single-minded and Contented to be Moderately Rich without any Wants." — NMV of Similitude 10:4, 13, and 25.

04-077 [_] "For the Remembrance of Evils, Works Death; but, the Forgetting of them, Works Eternal Life, which begins with Good Health." — NMV of Vision 1:23.

04-078 [_] "They are such as have Heard the Words of Truths, and were Willing to be Baptized in the Name of the Anointed Savior; but, after Considering the Great HOLINESS that the Truth

Requires, they have Withdrawn themselves from the Pursuit of it, and Walk again after their own Wicked Lusts, whereby they Seek Self-destruction without Knowing it." — NMV of Vision 3:76

04-079 [_] "From Faith proceeds Abstinence; from Abstinence, Simplicity; from Simplicity, Innocence; from Innocence, Modesty; from Modesty, Self-discipline; and from Self-discipline, Charity …"

04-080 [_] "For some People, by too free Feeding, contract an Infirmity in their Flesh, and do Injury to their Bodies; while the Flesh of others, who do not have Enough Foods, withers away: because they lack Sufficient Nourishment, and thus their Bodies are Consumed away by Hunger." — Vision 1:90 and 98.

04-081 [_] "They therefore that Repent Perfectly, shall be YOUNG in Body and Mind; and they who Turn from all of their Sins with their Whole Hearts, shall be Established on the Solid Bedrock of Divine Truths." — NMV of Vision 3:131.

04-082 [_] "Woe to the Doubtful Ones — to those Careless People, who shall Hear these Inspired Words of Provable Truths, and shall Despise them: because it had been Better for them, if they had not been Born." — NMV of Vision 4:22.

04-083 [_] "Especially see that you do not Speak Evil of anyone, nor Willingly Hear anyone Speak Evil of anyone else." (NOTE: That does Contradict several Scriptures, which most definitely Speak Evil of Evil People.)

04-084 [_] "Give without Distinction to all who are in Need, not Doubting to whom you Give. But, Give to all — even as God has Generously Given to all of us his own Good Gifts. Moreover, they who Receive our Gifts shall give an Account thereof to God, both for the Reason they Received, and for what they Do with the Things that they Receive. And they who Receive without a Real Need, shall give an Account for it; but, he who Gives shall be Innocent — even as God is Innocent, though he Gives to all of us his Blessings." — Command 2:2, and 6—8.

04-085 [_] "… And therefore I say to you, if anyone shall be Tempted by the Devil, and then Sin — after he has Obtained that Great and Holy Calling — he has but ONE Repentance. And if he shall often Sin, and Repent of it, it shall not Profit such a Person: because he shall hardly Live unto God." — Command 4:22.

04-086 [_] "Abstain therefore from all Evil, and you shall Know all Righteousness …" "Despise it therefore, and you shall always Rule over it on every Occasion."

04-087 [_] "But DOUBTING will not Believe, and therefore it shall not Obtain any Good Thing — not even by all that it can Do." — Command 8:2; and 9:9.

04-088 [_] "But, they who have the Fear of the Ruler in them, and Search out the Truth concerning the Supreme Ruler — having all of their Thoughts toward the Anointed One — Apprehend whatever is said to them, and forthwith Understand it: because they have the Reverence of the Anointed Savior within them." — Command 10:13.

04-089 [_] "When a Doubtful Man is Engaged in any Affair, and does not Accomplish it — by Reason of his Doubting — the Spirit of Sadness Enters into him, and Grieves the Holy Spirit, and that makes him Sad." — Command 10:15.

04-090 [_] "First of all, it is an Evil Desire to Covet another Man's Wife; or for a Wombman to have Longing Desires for another's Husband; as also to Desire the Dainties of Riches — even the Multitude of Superfluous Foods, as well as Drunkenness, and many Delights and Pleasures of the Flesh; because, in much Delicacy there is Folly; and many Pleasures are Needless to the Servants of God … For that Evil Lusting is DEADLY. You shall therefore put on the Desires of Righteousness and Holiness — being Armed with the Reverence of the Anointed One, Resisting all Wicked Lusting, Greed, Envy, Hate, and every Evil Spirit." — Command 12:4—6.

04-091 [_] "Put therefore, you who are Empty and Light in the Faith, the Anointed One, your Supreme Ruler, in your Hearts and Minds; and you shall Perceive how that nothing is more EASY than Obeying these Commands, nor more Pleasant, nor more Gentle and Holy." — Command 12:21.

04-092 [_] "I would therefore that you should now Do those Good Things, yourself, which in your Instructions you have Prescribed to others." — Romans 1:9 in the Lost Books of the Bible

04-093 [_] "I take no Pleasure in the Foods that Produce Corruption, nor in the Vain Pleasures of this Life — I Desire nothing but the Sweet Fruits from the Tree of Life, and the Peace that comes from the Supreme Ruler, only." — Romans 3:4, LBB (See Verse 04-092)

04-094 [_] "Also Pray without Ceasing for other Men: because there is Hope of Repentance in them, that they may Obtain unto a Godly State of Mind and Body: because they have not Sinned against such Great Nolij as you have; and, if God can Forgive you, he can also Forgive them. And let your Naaberz at least be Instructed by your Good Works, if they cannot be Instructed otherwise."

04-095 [_] "For the Beginning is Faith, and the End is Charity, which is the Pure Love of All that is Good. And when those 2 are Joined Together by True Love for the Supreme Ruler, there is no Good Thing that you cannot Do; but, all other Things that concern a Holy Life are the Consequences of those 2 Things." — Ephesians 3:1, and 14, Lost Books of the Bible (LBB).

04-096 [_] "Go up to Gilead, and take Balm — O you Virgin, the Daughter of Egypt — but, in Vain shall you use many Medicines: beCause you shall not be Cured by them." — Jeremiah 46:11, Revised King James Version (RKJV).

04-097 [_] "There is One Great Physician, both Fleshly and Spiritually … even Jesus Christ our Lord." — Ephesians 2:7, LBB.

04-098 [_] "… The Lord has said, Though you should be Joined unto me — even in my very Bosom — and yet you do not Love nor Obey my Commandments, I will Cat you Off, and say to you: Depart from me, O you Workers of Iniquities!" — Second Clement 2:15.

04-099 [_] "And let not anyone among you say that this very Flesh is not Judged, neither Raised Up from the Dead. Consider this, O Doubter — in WHAT were you Saved, in WHAT did you Look Up, if not while you were in this Body of Flesh that you Love so much? We must, therefore, keep our Flesh as the Temple of God — being HOLY and UNDEFILED. For in like manner, as you were Called in the Flesh, so shall you come to the Judgment Day in the Flesh. Indeed, even our One and Only Lord Jesus Christ, who has Saved us, being first a Spirit, was made Flesh, and thus Dwelt among us, and so he Called us; even so we shall also Receive our Rewards while in our Flesh. Let us, therefore, Love one another with TRUE Love: so that we might Attain Positions in the Holy Kingdom of the Gods. Therefore, while we have Time to be Healed, let us Deliver ourselves up to our God, who is our Great Physician, giving our Reward and Praise to him {rather than Paying the Doctor Knife for Services that were not Needed}. And what Reward shall we give? — Repentance from a Pure Heart: because he Knows all Things before they are at Hand, and he Searches out our very Bowels." — NMV of Second Clement 4:1—4, LBB.

04-100 [_] "For if we shall do our Diligence to Live Well during this Life, Peace will Follow us. And yet how Difficult it is to Find a single Man on the Earth who Does that: because almost all are Led by Human Fears, Choosing the Present Enjoyments and Vain Pleasures, rather than the Future Promises with Fathers Abraham, Isaac, and Jacob; but, they Know not how Great a Torment that the Present Enjoyments bring with them, nor what Great DELIGHTS that the Future Promises shall bring to us who Love and Obey all of the Laws of the Supreme Ruler." — Second Clement 4:7—8, LBB.

04-101 [_] "Beloved, the Reproof and the Correction, which we Exercise towards one another, is Good, and Exceedingly Profitable: because it Unites us the more Closely with the Will of our Supreme Ruler." — First Clement 23:4, LBB.

04-102 [_] "Let him who is Pure in the Flesh, not grow PROUD of it — Knowing that it was from another that he Received the Gift of Continence." — First Clement 17:38, LBB.

04-103 [_] "Let our Praise be of God only, not of ourselves: because God Hates those People who Commend themselves, as if they had Done or could Do something Great without the Assistance of their Creator." — NMV of First Clement 14:7.

04-104 [_] "O you Fools! — consider the Fruit Trees — Look at the Grapevine for a Good Example. First it Sheds its Leaves, then it Fasts all Winter, and then it Buds; after that it Spreads its Leaves, and then it Flowers; and then come the Sour Grapes; and after that Follows the Sweet Ripe Fruits … according to the Cycles of Life and Death, which are one Eternal Round, Year in, and Year out: because all Trees and Vines are Regenerated each Year, when they Rest." — NMV of First Clement 11:13, LBB. {NOTE: Many Trees are Evergreens, whereby they Lose a few Leaves at a Time, which is like Shedding Skin.}

04-105 [_] "Let us Search into all of the Ages, which have gone before us, and let us Learn that our Lord has been Merciful in every one of them, and has still given a Time for Repentance to all such People as would Turn to him. For Example, Noah Preached Repentance, and as many as Listened to him were Saved with a Temporal Salvation. Jonah also Pronounced Destruction against the Ninevites; howbeit, they Repented of their Sins, Appeasing the Wrath of God by their Fastings and Prayers; and were thus Saved from Destruction — even though they were complete Strangers to the Covenants of our God!" — NMV of First Clement 4:6—8, LBB.

04-106 [_] "Therefore, let us Humble ourselves by Means of Fasting and Praying, Brothers — while laying aside all Pride, Boasting, Foolishness, and Anger — and let us do as it is Written. For thus says the Holy Spirit: Let not the Wise Man Glory in his Wisdom, nor the Strong Man in his Strength, nor the Rich Man in his Riches; but, let him who Glories, Glory in the Supreme Ruler, to Seek him, and to Do Judgment with Justice for all. And above all, Remember the Words of the Lord Jesus, which he Spoke concerning EQUITY and LONG SUFFERING, saying: Be you Merciful and you shall Obtain Mercy; Forgive, and you shall be Forgiven; as you Do, so shall it be Done unto you, sooner or later, either during this Life or the next Life; indeed, as you Give, so shall it be Given unto you; as you Judge, so shall you be Judged; as you are Kind to others, so shall God be Kind to you: because with what Measure that you Measure with, with the same shall it be Measured to you again, sooner or later, either during this Life, or during the Life to come: because all Spirits are Recycled, over and over, until they are brought to Perfection for either Good or Evil. Therefore, by that Command, and by these Rules, let us Establish ourselves so that we may always Walk Obediently to his Holy Words — being Humble-minded: beCause so says the Scriptures — Upon whom shall I Look with Favors? — even upon him who is Poor and of a Contrite Spirit, and who Trembles at the Sound of my Words of Truths." — NMV of First Clement 7:1.

04-107 [_] "You see, Beloved Brothers, what the Pattern is that has been Given to us? For if the Lord thus Humbled himself by Means of Fasting and Praying, what should we Do, who are brought by him under the Yoke of his Grace? Let us be Followers of those who went about in Goat Skins and Sheep Skins, Preaching the Coming of Christ, and the Glory of his Great Kingdom, which is Composed of Holy People, who are Perfected in his own Image." — NMV of First Clement 8:16, LBB.

04-108 [_] "The Spirit of the Lord is like a Candle — Searching out the Inwards Parts of the Belly and Mind."

04-109 [_] "Let us Choose to Offend a few Foolish and Inconsiderate Men, who are lifted up in their Pride, and Glorying in their own Abilities, rather than Offend the Creator, who is Able to Destroy both our Bodies and Spirits like Trash that is thrown into a Fire."

04-110 [_] "Let the Government o four Tongues be made Known by our SILENCE."

04-111 [_] "And especially let us Learn how Great a Power that Humility has with God; how much a Pure and Holy Charity Avails with him; how Excellent and Great his Fear is; and how it will Save all such People as Turn to him in Holiness with a Pure Mind." — NMV of First Clement 10:2, 5, 10, and 13, LBB.

04-112 [_] "… insomuch that the Physicians of Seleucia were now of no more Account or Use, and lost all of the Profit from the Sale of their Craft: because no one Regarded them, nor Bought their Drugs, whereupon the Physicians were filled with Envy, and began to contrive what

Methods to Use, in Order to get Rid of this Servant of Christ, who Taught Fasting and Praying as a Remedy for all Ailments." — NMV of Paul and Thecia 10:18, LBB.

04-113 [_] "… Thus with Violence shall that huge City of Confusion be thrown down, and shall not be found any more at all … and no Craftsman, of whatever Craft he is, shall be found anymore in you … for by your Druggeries were all of the Nations on the Earth Deceived." — Revelation 18, RKJV.

04-114 [_] "And after that, I Repented with a Set Purpose of my Soul for SEVEN YEARS in front of the Lord. And neither Wine nor Strong Drinks did I Drink; and Flesh did not Enter into my Mouth; and I Ate no Pleasant Foods; but, I Mourned over my Sin: because it was so Great, such as had not been in Israel." — Reuben 1, in the Forgotten Books of Eden (FBE).

04-115 [_] "Therefore, for 2 Years I Afflicted my Soul by Means of Fasting in the Fear of the Lord …" — Simeon 1:18, FBE.

04-116 [_] "For the Devil is eager to Destroy all People who call on the Lord: because he Knows that upon the Day in which Israel shall Repent, the Kingdom of the Enemy shall be brought to an End!" — Daniel 2:16—17, LBB.

04-117 [_] "And I Fasted during those Seven Years, and I Appeared to the Egyptians as one living delicately, for they that Fast for God's Sake receive Beauty of Face." — Joseph 1:29, FBE

04-118 [_] "… Now I would that you should Remember that God has said that the INWARD VESSEL shall be CLEANSED FIRST, and then shall the Outer Vessel be Clean also." — Alma 60:23.

04-119 [_] "And there shall arise in the Latter Days one who is Beloved of the Lord, of the Tribe of Judah and Levi — even a Doer of his Good Pleasure in his Mouth, with new Nolij, Enlightening the Gentiles — until the Consummation of the Ages, shall he be in the Synagogues of the Gentiles, and among their Rulers, as a Strain of Music in the Mouths of all who Hear his Inspired Words of Provable Truths. Moreover, he shall be Inscribed in the Holy Books, both for his Works and for his Words, and he shall be a Chosen One of God Forever …" — NMV of Benjamin 2:26—29, FBE.

04-120 [_] And those are just SOME of many Words of Truths that were Disgracefully LEFT OUT of the *"Holy Bible."* Moreover, to make Matters Worse, many Words were Mistranslated. For Example, "Fruits" are called "Bread," which should have been Translated as "Food" or "Foods," instead of Bread, throughout the Bible. However, by Translating it "Bread," we now Know for a Fact that it is "speaking" of the FRUITS, which is really Great Nolij, which most Bibles do not contain. Moreover, the Water of Life is the JUICE that is found within those Sweet Juicy Fruits. Therefore, to Eat the Bread of Life, and to Drink the Water of Life, means to Eat the Sweet Juicy Fruits from the Tree of Life. Indeed, there is no other Rational Explanation for such Symbolical Words that are BOTH Temporal AND Spiritual!

— Chapter 05 —

Other Reasons and Persuasive Arguments in Favor of Fasting

05-01 [_] Most People are Ignorant concerning the Facts about Fasting and the Great Benefits that Fasting has for every Person who Practices it according to **"The Proper RULES for FASTING!"** even if they do not Believe any of those Ancient Sacred Writings in any Versions that are "Quoted" in the Previous Chapter, which I have Enhanced to a certain Limited Degree, just to make Sure that the Words are Plain and Easy to Understand, even as I have done with the entire *Bible, the Apocrypha, the Book of Mormon, the Koran, the Lost Books of the Bible,* and *the Forgotten Books of Eden,* with the Hope that at least someone might Appreciate it. However, most Silly People are not the Slightest Bit Interested in TRUTHS; but, they are Greatly Concerned with whether or not the Words were "translated correctly from the original languages," as if that were even Possible, let alone Practical: beCause, who would read very much of a Book that was written Backwards, Upside Down, and without any Vowels? Yes, that would be Original Hebrew. Yes, Hbrw th rgnl tht wld b, and Upside Down and Backwards.

05-02 [_] A True Christian would not even be Looking for Meaningless Faults, lest he or she should Miss the Message. Indeed, a True Christian would be Looking for TRUTHS, and even Provable Truths, which can Stand Up in a Courtroom, and WIN the Case. Such is the Case for all Truths about all Subjects. For Example, I will now Quote to you from *the Gospel According to Saint John Zebedee Boanerges,* who relates what Jesus Christ Revealed about Fasting, which is most Enlightening to our Minds: because it is so Crystal Clear, like the Brightness of the Sunlight on a Clear Cloudless Day. Therefore, please be very Patient: because there is nothing so Precious as the Truth, even if that Truth was Revealed thousands of Years Ago. After all, the Nature of Mankind, and the Construction of the Human Body has not Changed since the Beginning, as all Honest Scientists Agree. Indeed, the CURE for most of our Ailments, as well as those of Animals, is Basically FASTING: because it is Nature's one and ONLY Sure Cure or Remedy for Dietary Sins, without which Nature has nothing to Offer: because no Amount of Medicines can CURE a BAD HABIT, nor Eliminate an ADDICTION; but, Fasting can Do it, and you can easily Prove it, just by Practicing it According to **"The Complete Instruction Manual for True Repentance!"** Therefore, please be Patient, until we get around to those most Important Rules, in my Inspired Book, called: **"The Proper RULES for FASTING!"** — some of which should be Memorized and Meditated on.

05-03 [_] Indeed, after that, Yoshua (which is the Hebrew Name for the Savoir, which was Translated as "Jesus," in English, comes from the Greek ZEUS, who was the Supreme God in Greek Mythology, which is pronounced Haa-sqs in Spanish, for Example, is a Perversion of the Hebrew Meaning, even though there are Similarities: because both "Gods" were Saviors and Supreme Rulers) went down to Capernaum {pronounced Ku-PER-naw-um}, which is a Palestinian Name, which means Village by the Sea; and he went with his Disciples, who were now very much in Love with him, as well as his Mother and Brothers, who also went with him;

but, they did not stay in Capernaum very long: because most of the People were Wealthy and Proud, and did not Accept our Anointed Savior: because they Trusted in their False Riches to Save them. Yes, they Believed in Baal to Save them, which is the God of Possessions. Moreover, they did not Believe the Rumors that they had Heard about the Miracles in Cana of Galilee: because of those Lying Servants, who could not always be Trusted to the Tell the Whole Truth.

05-04 [_] Nevertheless, there was a Sick Lad there, who had Eaten some Spoiled Food, and was in Great Pains, whom Yoshqu {spelled in Funetik Ingglish} Touched as he passed by, and the Lad was Instantly Healed: because Yoshqu had Power to Heal the Sick People, as well as Animals who got Injured. However, most of the People said that it was just another Magician's Trick: because some said that he had given the Boy something to Eat, which they Credited with the Power to Heal him; but, others said that he had not given to him anything to Eat; but, that he had only Touched him.

05-05 [_] Therefore, a few People began to Believe on him; but, not with all of their Hearts. No, they could not Accept him as their Anointed Savior: because they were not Taught the *Scriptures,* even as we were Taught by our Parents; and therefore, they did not have any Good Foundation on which to Build their Faith: because the Seeds of Truths had not been Sown in their Hearts when they were just Children, whereby they might have Sprouted and Grown and Nourished them along. No, they had not Learned so much as the Inspired Writings of Moses: because they were too Busy with their own Worldly Ambitions, and did not take the Time to Learn the Important Lessons of Life; and therefore, they all Suffered with Various Kinds of Ailments, with Aches and Pains, both Day and Night; but, they still would not Believe in the Messiah, who is their Anointed Savior: beCause they had no Faith in him, and could not bring themselves around to Believe his Inspired Words of Lovable Truths, which he Tried to Teach to them, saying:

05-06 [_] How Long will you People Suffer in your States of Ignorance and Pride? Do you not Know that every Body was Created in such a Way as to Heal itself? Indeed, no Wild Animals have any Doctors, Nurses, Hospitals, Drug Stores, nor even a Book from which to Learn the Truth about any Subject; but, if they get Sick or Badly Wounded, they Instinctively Know what do about it: because they simply Lose their Appetites, whereby they Stop Eating and Drinking; but, you People have entire Libraries, full of all Kinds of Vain books, which contain False knowledge, or else you would be Able to Learn the Truth, and thus be Healed from your Ailments; but, behold, you are Suffering with Various Kinds of Sicknesses and Diseases, for which there is no Remedy without True Nolij, Faith, Hope, Trust, Patience, Love, and Obedience to certain Divine and Natural Laws of the Gods — that is, of the Great Family of Holy Ones who Created the Heavens and the Earths without Number, being Countless to any Man, who could not Live Long Enough to Count even one-millionth of them.

05-07 [_] Therefore, Exercise your Faith, since you Know that I Healed the Lad, who now sits at the Doorway of this House, who Truly Believes in me: because I made him Well, and you can See that his Eyes are Sparkling with Delight, just to Hear my Inspired Words of Provable Truths; but, those same Words have no Benefit whatsoever to those People who are Hardhearted, who Close their Spiritual Ears, who Refuse to Believe and be Saved from all of their Sins and Woes: because their Spiritual Ears are Filled with the Wax of Unbelief; and therefore, they cannot even

Hear the Words. Moreover, their Eyes are Covered with Scales of Slime, so that they cannot See: because they are Blinded by their Great Pride, which is very Blinding to the Mind of Man: because the Spirit of Pride is of the Devil, who uses it to Blind our Minds.

05-08 [_] Therefore, let us Humble ourselves, and Confess that there is only One Way for us to Escape from the Prison of Pride, which is to Pass Through the Doorway of Confession, which Requires Humility of Mind, just in Order to Discover the KEY of True Nolij concerning All that is Good and Evil, which Key can be Used Wisely to Unlock the Door of Confession, which Prevents us from Escaping from the Prison of Lies.

05-09 [_] Indeed, you have lots of word knowledge in your Public Libraries, and you have Eyes that can See those words; but, you need Truth Nolij: because word knowledge, alone, cannot Save you; but, it will only PUFF UP your Minds with BLINDING PRIDE, and thus make you Imagine that you are Wise, even if you are little more than the Lowest Class Ignorant Fools on this Earth! Yes, you are like little Children, who go to some School of Fools, and learn a few Words, and come back Home Imagining that they Know more than their own Parents!

05-10 [_] Therefore, Humble yourselves, and Confess that you are Lacking MANY Great Truths that you Need to Learn, in Order to Escape from that Prison of Pride and Blinding Lies, into which you were Born, and could not Help yourselves. But, behold, there is a little Light of Truth Shining through your Window of Faith, if it is not Covered Up with those Dark Curtains of Doubt and Unbelief, which Light is Revealing the KEY of the Nolij of ALL that is Good and Evil to you, if you Look for it, which is Hidden in the Darkness of Ignorance, among all of those Countless books on Nonsense, which are a Waste of your Precious Time to Study.

05-11 [_] Yes, I Realize that it is your Vain Tradition to Cook Various Kinds of Foods, and to Stuff yourselves with Various Mixtures of Tempting Concoctions, and to make yourselves Sick by Eating Swine's Flesh and whatever Dead Carcasses you can drag Home; but, the True Foods for Mankind are the Sweet Ripe Juicy RAW Fresh Fruits from the Trees of Life, which are found in Abundance in the Blest Land of Perfect Oneness, in the Paradise of Peace and True Happiness, which is the Fruitful Garden of the Great King, whose Humble Children are those who Obey his Voice, who Love his Inspired Words of Provable Truths, who have Tried the Experiment of Fasting and Praying, combined with certain Days of Feasting on those Sweet Juicy Fruits, which most of you People would not Dare to Do: beCause your Bowels are Filled with Excess FILTH, which would Cause you to Vomit, or perhaps even Cause you to Die from Gasses and Cramps within your Bowels: because of the Fermentation that would be Caused by those Sweet Fruits being Mixed with Various Kinds of Ancient Morbid Matter.

05-12 [_] Therefore, you must Humble yourselves, and DENY yourselves of those Foods that Cause you to become so Constipated and Sick. Yes, you must Deny yourselves of any Fleshly Lusts, while Remembering the Children of Israel, who Lusted after Flesh in the Wilderness, and who Died in a Great Plague, according to *Numbers 11;* and you must Try to Live on Natural Wholesome Foods, until your Bowels are Working more like mine, which are not Constipated: because you can See that I do not Appear to be Pregnant, as many of you Men do: because your Bellies are hanging on your Neez, you might say, which Means that your Internal Pipe Systems are CLOGGED UP, just like your Sink Drains and Toilet Drains, which are Filled with Greasy

Filth, which comes from your own Kitchens: because you Love those Greasy Fried Foods, and are not Ashamed of Feasting with the Hogs and Dogs, who have no Discretion, who cannot Discern what is Good and what is Evil for them: because they are Accustomed to such Vain Traditions; but, now you Know that it is a SIN for him to Eat that which he Knows for a Fact is NO GOOD for him.

05-13 [_] Yes, it is a Sin for any Person to do anything that he or she Knows within himself or herself is WRong: because Nature itself Teaches to us what is Riit and Rong, and we will do Well to Accept our Lessons from Nature: because Nature has all Kinds of Good Examples for us to Learn from.

05-14 [_] Indeed, we can be like Sheeps and Cows, or else we can be like Goats and Asses; but, many People Willfully Choose to be like Hogs and Bears, who can get as Fat as Tubs of Lard, and still not Confess that something must be wRong with their Diets. Yes, something must be WRong with their SPIRITUAL Eating Habits: beCause their Thinking is WRong: beCause of Lusting after that which is Forbidden, which is WHY that they have an Appetite to Consume Various Kinds of Abominations, which only the Deceived Rich People could even Afford to Buy. Therefore, Blest are those Poor Hungry Souls, who have not Stuffed themselves with so much Pride and so many Lies, who can Understand my Inspired Words of Provable Truths. Amen.

05-15 [_] And with those Words, Yoshqu finished his Speech, which Caused many of those Deceived Rich People to become very Angry: because they were put to Shame for their Evil Habits, which also Caused most of them to get Red Ears: because his Words of Truths were very Embarrassing to them: because they were Guilty of Gluttony and Drunkenness, and they Knew that they were doing WRong to Live according to the Manner of those Hogs and Bears, who Glut themselves: because it is not Necessary that People should Glut themselves, since People can Store Foods for the Winter Months, inside of Buildings, and in Canning Jars, whereby they Eat whenever they Need to Eat; but, Bears like to Sleep all Winter, and therefore it is no Sin for them to Feast all Summer: because they have to Store Up Fat for the Winter; but, People only need a Small Amount of Fat, in order to Maintain Good Health.

05-16 [_] Nevertheless, those Inspired Words of Provable Truths were too much for those Capernaumites to Accept, or to even Try to Prove to be Right or WRong: beCause they were not Willing to Experiment with his Words, and Humble themselves by Means of Fasting; but, they were only Highly Offended by his Words, even as any Guilty Person is Offended by the Truths that might be Revealed about him. No, they would not Fast nor Pray for even one Day, nor Change their Diets in any Way: because they were Fully Persuaded that their Traditional Way of Living was Correct, and that it is no Sin to Eat nor Drink so much: because their Cattle Feasted on Grasses all Day Long, except to Chew on their Cuds; and their Hogs would Eat anything that was set in front of them, which they Assumed was Good for them.

05-17 [_] However, something was WRong: because they Suffered with Various Kinds of Sicknesses and Diseases, which is WHY that Yoshqu Tried to Enlighten their Minds; but, they Hardened their Hearts against him, and Refused to Accept him as their Anointed Savior; and therefore, he Departed from them, and left them to Suffer.

05-18 [_] Now, there was a certain Man of the Sect of the Pharisees, named Nicodemus, a Ruler among the Jews, who came to the Anointed Savior during the Night, in Secret, and said to him: "Master, we Know that you are a Teacher, who has come from God: because no Man can Do all of the Miracles that you Do, except that our God is with him. Therefore, I am now Wondering HOW that I could get the Gifts that you have?"

05-19 [_] Yoshua Answered him, "Truly, Truly, I say to you: Except a Man is Born Again, he cannot even See nor Understand the Kingdom of the Supreme Ruler." Therefore, Nicodemus said to him, "How can a Man be Born Again when he is Old — can he Enter into his Mother's Womb for the Second Time, and be Born Again? Do you Accept the Doctrine of those People who Live in the East, in India, who say that we have all Lived before: because it is Impossible for a Person to Learn all of his or her Lessons during only one Lifetime; and therefore, it Requires many Lives, in Order to Learn all such Lessons?"

05-20 [_] Yoshua Answered, "Truly, Truly, I say to you: Except a Man is Born of Water, and is also Born of the Spirit, he cannot Enter into the Kingdom of the Most High Ruler, which is a Great Pyramid Government, with the Most High Ruler at the very Top of it, being the Golden Capstone, himself, who is the Invisible God, whom no Man has ever Seen: because he is a Great Spirit Being, who also Controls Seven Great Spirits, one of which is the Holy Spirit, who brings all Things back to our Remembrance, once we have Learned those Things. Therefore, I am telling you that each Spirit of each Man must be Tested for its Goodness, before it can Qualify to Enter into that Holy Kingdom of All that is Good, which is God. Indeed, they who are Born of the Flesh are Flesh and Blood, who are Born by Water from the Womb; but, they who are Born of the Spirit are Spiritual: because the Heavenly Father Adopts them into his Holy Family of Spiritual Beings, who have One Mind, One Understanding, One Opinion, One Agreement, One Great Hope, One Faith, One Baptism by Fire, and One True Love — who all Love each other as a True United Family of Holy Ones. Therefore, do not Marvel that I said to you, that you must be Born Again: because all People must be Born Again of Water and Spirit, before they can Enter into the Holy Kingdom of the Most High Ruler, unless they are Perfected during this Lifetime, in which Case they will not have to Live Again, until the Resurrection: because they have Passed their Tests of Nolij, Faith, Hope, Trust, Patience, Love, and Obedience. Indeed, the Wind Blows wherever it Desires to go, and you can Hear the Sound that it Makes; but, you cannot tell where it comes from, nor where it is going to. Likewise, so is every Person who is Born of the Spirit, which comes like the Wind, which Transforms the Mind of Man, and makes him like a New Creature: because Old Things are passed Away, and behold, all Things are NEW: because he who Humbles himself by Means of much Fasting and Praying, and Confesses all of his Sins, and Cleanses himself from all Filthiness of his Mind and Body, is Purged from all Uncleanness from Head to Toe, and is therefore Physiologically and Spiritually Born Again: because he is Filled with the Holy Spirit, which can only Live within Clean Temples. Nevertheless, that Spirit can Visit any Temple for a Short Time, even if it is Unclean: because she Draws People to our Heavenly Father, who Lives Inside of Jupiter, who is called Yohoovu or Jehovah God. Therefore, if People only Sincerely Confess all of their Sins, and Repent to that Degree, they are Blest with a Portion of his Holy Spirit: because he must let them Know that he Loves them for whatever Goodness might be within them. Therefore, his Holy Spirit Enters into them for a certain Length of Time, just to let them Know that they are Headed in the Right Direction, even if they have Perverse Religious Beliefs, like those People of India, who Vainly Imagine that

People can become Cattle, Rats, or even Dogs and Snakes. Nevertheless, they cannot have the Fullness of his Holy Spirit, until they are Holy, even as I am Holy, which Means that they must be Pure in Mind and Body, even as I am Pure: because I am your Good Example, who can also do Miracles, in Order to Prove it."

05-21 [_] And Nicodemus said to him, "How can those things be? How can the Holy Spirit Judge who is Worthy of her Spirit, and who is not Worthy? Are not all Children Born Holy? Must they also Repent by Means of Fasting and Praying, as you say, in Order to be Saved for some Positions within the Kingdom of the Gods, who might even Inherit their very own Worlds?" And Yoshua Answered him, "Are you a Master of Israel, and do not Know those Basic Truths? Did John the Baptist not Teach to you all of those Good Lessons? Truly, Truly, I say to you: We Speak of that which we do Know for a Fact, and we Testify of that which we have Seen; and yet you Scribes and Pharisees do not Accept our Witness to those Great Truths: because you have not Fasted nor Earnestly Prayed for Forgiveness for ALL of your Sins, including your Dietary Sins, which Prevent you from Understanding my Inspired Words of Provable Truths. However, if I have told you about Earthly Things, and you do not Believe that Good News, how shall you Believe, if I tell you about Heavenly Things? And Remember this, NO Man has Ascended up to Heaven at any Time, to the Throne of the Most High Ruler, who does not even Live within this Galaxy, nor in this so-called Universe, which is just one of Multitudes of Universes, some of which are a million Times as large as this Universe: beCause there are Endless Creations, which go on and on for ever and ever! Nevertheless, the Son of the Man of Holiness, who Lives Inside of Jupiter, has Ascended up to that Heavenly Place: because he is the Selected KING of Kings of this World, who is also the Chosen Son of the Most High Ruler of this Galaxy, who Lives in a World in Orion, who Chose a certain Man called Joseph to Bear the Holy Seed from which I was Conceived within the Womb of a Holy Wombman, called Mary, by the Power of the Holy Spirit, which came upon my Parents while they Slept, before they had Sexual Intercourse: because it was Appointed to them to be Blest with a Holy Child, who would be the Savior of the People of the World, to as many as will Accept him and Obey his Inspired Words of Provable Truths.

05-22 [_] "Indeed, as Moses Lifted Up the Brass Serpent in the Wilderness, so that all Men who had been Bitten by any Poisonous Serpents might Look on it, and be Saved Alive, even so the Son of a certain Man must be Lifted Up on a Torture Stake: so that everyone can be Saved from their Sins by Means of his Sufferings for them, whose Minds have been Poisoned by that Sly Old Serpent, called the Devil, who has Successfully Deceived almost all Peoples on the Earth. Nevertheless, whosoever Believes in the Son of a certain Man, and Obeys his Lovable Words of Divine Truths, will not Perish; but, will have Everlasting Good Health: because I am come so that you might have Good Health, and have it more Abundantly: because the Supreme Ruler Loved the People of the World so much, that he Gave his only Son, who was Begotten by the Power of the Holy Spirit, so that whosoever Truly and Sincerely Believes in him should not Perish, even as they did not Perish when Moses were here; but, they shall have Everlasting Good Health, which is also Everlasting Life, which Begins with Good Health: because the Supreme Ruler did not Send his Son into the World, in Order to Condemn the People of the World; but, so that the People of the World might be Saved through Faith in him, by his Grace and Mercy, by Humble Obedience to his Words of Truths: because, without Grace and Mercy, there was no Binding Promise that he should Come, nor even Teach anyone anything about Life, Love,

Happiness, nor any Good Thing: because all of those Good Things come beCause of Grace and Mercy: because our Heavenly Father is Full of Grace and Mercy: because of his Great Love for his Children, which is Revealed by his Only Begotten Son.

05-23 [ ] "Therefore, he who Believes on him who was Sent to Save them, is not Condemned; but, he who does not Believe in him, is Condemned already: because he has not Believed in the Name of the Only Son who was Begotten by the Power of the Holy Spirit. Moreover, this is the Condemnation, that Light and Truths have come into the World; but, Unclean People have Loved the Darkness of Ignorance more than the Light of Truths: beCause their Thoughts and Deeds are Evil. Indeed, everyone who does Evil, HATES the Light of Truths; and will not come into the Light, lest his Evil Deeds should be Discovered, and his Sins Exposed; but, he who does Good, LOVES the Light of Truths, and therefore Gladly comes into the Light: so that his Good Deeds might be made Known, that they are Worked According to the Will of the Supreme Ruler, who would have all People to Do Good Works, rather than to Do Evil Works: because there is no Profit nor Gain by Doing Evil Works: because Evil Breeds more and more Evils, until at last all of the People are Suffering under the Tyrannical Domain of an Evil Empire, which makes Tax Slaves, Usury Slaves, Insurance Slaves, Drug Slaves, and Work Slaves of those Unwise Ignorant People, who could simply Learn, Believe, Love, and Obey the Laws of the Master Farmer, and be FREE from all such Slavery; but, instead, they Willingly Choose to Do Evil, whereby they get their Just Rewards. And now, to Answer your Question, 'Are not all Children Born Holy?' you can See that they are NOT: because, if they were, they would be like me; but, instead, some of them are like little Demons: because they are Born from Unholy Parents. Indeed, each Tree Produces Fruits like itself, according to its Health."

05-24 [ ] Then Nicodemus Interrupted his Speech, and said to Yoshua, "Are you saying that a Good Government would not have any Taxes? If so, WHO would Pay for the Services of Government Officials and their Armies?" And Yoshua Answered him, "Truly, Truly, I say to you, that a Righteous GovernMint would simply Mint the Necessary Silver and Gold Coins, in Order to Use that New Money Wisely, in Order to HIRE whomever is Willing and Able to Learn and Work, in Order to Help Build their own Beautiful Stone Dome Homes, Home-craft Workshops, Fruit Tree Houses, Stone Walls, Tunnels, Cisterns, Stairways, and whatever they Need for True Prosperity at Home, including large Gardens, which should be Directly in Front of their Houses, which should be Built in large Terraces: so that all Roofs are Covered with Gardens: so that no Space is Wasted; and that Stonework will Represent that New Money, which must be Earned by Honest Labor, without any Loans, without any Usury, and without any Taxes, with all Men being Paid EQUAL WAGES for EQUAL SERVICES, which will make that Money just as Valuable as the Effort that it is Required to Earn it; and therefore, everyone within that Righteous Kingdom can Obtain their own Beautiful Stone Dome Home Complex, if they are Willing and Able to Learn and Work, which includes almost all People.

05-25 [ ] "Nevertheless, there is no Need for each Family Owning their own Stone Dome Home Complex: because, if they were Willing to Work to Build it, they should be Able to Live in it, Rent-free, until they Die, at which Time their Children can Inherit it, along with whatever Houses and Gardens that they have Built, which should all be Constructed in a Permanent Way: so as to Endure the Test of Time: beCause this World is our Eternal Home, which we should take Good Care of: because it is all that we have to Work with. Moreover, when all of the People

Learn to Love and Obey ALL of my Commandments, there will be NO Stealing, NO Murdering, NO Raping, NO Robbing, and thus no Need for Collecting any Taxes to Maintain Law and Order: because all of those Wise People will LOVE their Leaders, and will therefore Cheerfully Support them with Freewill Offerings and Donations, as well as Help them to Build their own Palaces, which will Belong to the Masses of People: because there are very few Officials Needed within such a Righteous Kingdom, which does not Need to Maintain any Army of Defenders: because WHO can Overcome People who are Living in Well-Fortified City States, if they are Built Properly, which have all of the Gardens, Vineyards, Orchards, Houses, Cisterns, and Home-craft Workshops and Sales Shops within the Borders of their STRONG Fortified Planned City States? Yes, WHO can Afford to Attack them and Overcome them, once they are well Dug in, with lots of Tunnels, large Moats full of Running Water, millions of large Cisterns, and whatever Stone Walls and Steel Gates that they Need to Defend themselves? Truly, Truly, I say to you, only a General fool would even Contemplate such an Attack: beCause it would be Futile and Self-defeating: because no such Fortified City can be Overcome by any Small Means, and it is certainly not Worth the Great Expense of Trying to Overcome it, when any Group of Wise People could go to Work and Build their own Beautiful Planned City State, with the Help of Mechanical Beasts, which might do the Work of thousands of Strong Young Men, even as it will be during the Last Days. Therefore, the Wise People will Foresee the Evils that are Coming, and get themselves Prepared for the Worst: because it is Possible for the Worst Things to Happen to them, just in Order to Test their Nolij, Skills, Abilities, Faith, Hope, Trust, Patience, Persistence, Love, and Obedience: because the Devil Rules over the Unholy Kingdoms of this World, and he Inspires some of them to Invent Evil Things, and to go to War: because he Loves those Gory Bloody Wars; but, WHO can make War against the Holy City of the Great King, which is Guarded by the Holy Angels, and which is Baptized continually with Flames of Devouring Fire from the Supreme Ruler, which would Consume any Trespassers?"

05-26 [_] And Nicodemus said to him, "Are you that Great King who is to come during these Last Days, in Order to Establish your Good Government over all Nations under the Sky; or, should we Look for someone else, and have Faith in some other Person, who might Speak more Plainly than yourself?" And Yoshua Answered him, "Truly, Truly, I say to you, that I was Born to be a Great King, who shall Rule all Nations with a Rod of Iron; but, not until I have Established my Kingdom within the Hearts and Minds of all Honest Men, who must Learn to Govern themselves, and to Conquer the Beastly Nature within themselves: because that is the Dreaded Enemy, which everyone should Fear the Most to Submit to: because, if that Beast is not Overcome, the Devil will have Rulership Over you, whereby all such Fortresses can be Destroyed from within. Therefore, let every Man Strive to Overcome all of his Sins, and to STOP Sinning: because it is Sin that Separates him from the Supreme Ruler, who will Establish his Holy Kingdom during these Last Days: because there is a Great Day of Peaceful Rest coming, even that Great Sabbath Day, which is the Seventh Day; but, be not Ignorant of this one Important Thing — that One Day to the Supreme Ruler is a Thousand Years, and a Thousand Years is One Day. Therefore, when Six Thousand Years have passed since the Beginning, when Adam and Eve were Cast Out of the Paradise of God, after they Sinned, I will Come to Govern the World; but, only IF my Bride is Ready. Yes, it is Based on the CONDITION that my Church has become Holy, even as I am Holy: because I will not Return for an Unholy Bride. Therefore, the Church of Christ must Do whatever it must Do to be Saved from all Sins, and to Overcome them, which can only be Possible if that Church Learns to Cooperate with the Truths that I

Teach, and to Build their own Beautiful Planned City State, which they may call the New Jerusalem, having no less than 6 Courts, whereby the People may Work their Way Toward the Innermost Court from the Outermost Court, which Innermost Court must be the Holiest of all Courts, which must be Supported by the other Courts, who See a Vision of what is Needed for Overcoming the Devil and his Multitude of Temptations, which will Surround them on all Sides. Yes, it calls for the Establishment of **'The New RIGHTEOUS One-World Government!'** Yes, there will be a Holy One-World Government during the Future, which will not Need any Money: because everyone will have True Love for everyone else; and therefore, all People will have all Things in Common among them, and they will Work in Unison, like a Team of Workhorses: so that they might all become Moderately Rich in all Ways: so that there will be no Poor People among them, nor any Extravagantly Rich People among them; but, they will Share their Wealth among all of the Righteous People, while Casting Out all of the Wicked Disobedient People from among them, who may Live with the Lions and Bears in the Wilderness, along with Snakes, Scorpions, Skunks, and whatever might Live out there. Therefore, before that Happy Day of Peaceful Rest for a Thousand Years, there will be a New Righteous One-World GovernMINT Established, which will Do what I said before, and will Mint and Print the Necessary New Money for HIRING **'Seven Great Armies of Working Soldiers,'** or whomever is Willing and Able to Learn and Work, in Order to Help Build those **'GLORIOUS Swanky Hotels Castles and Fortresses,'** which will make it Possible for them to Clean Up the Earth, and Stop Polluting it with their Abominations: because there will come a Time when Nolij shall be Greatly Increased, and this Good News will be Published to all Peoples in all Nations: because it is Necessary to Save those Wise People who will Believe and Obey my Inspired Words of Provable Truths."

05-27 [ ] And Nicodemus said to him, "You Speak with Riddles, O Master House Builder, which no one can Understand. Indeed, are you saying that you will Live for another 3,000 Years!?" And Yoshua said to him, "Are you a Master in Israel, and do not Know the Scriptures? Truly, Truly, I say to you, the Master House Builder of this World will be Judged and Condemned by the Scribes and Pharisees, who are Descendants of Esau, who have taken over the Temple Services, and have Administered their own False Doctrines to these Ignorant People, while also Establishing Banks and Bankers, who no longer Believe in the Holy Kingdom of the Gods, much less that they might Qualify for any such Positions within that Great Kingdom, whereby they might Inherit their very own Worlds, if they Prove themselves to be Worthy of it in this World, which, of course, less than one Man in a Billion has ever Accomplished; but, there are many Offices to be Fulfilled, even for that one who does Qualify, who will Naturally Need his Administration with many Servants. Therefore, it is a Worthy Goal to Strive for, which has its own Good Rewards, even if one does not Succeed in becoming such a Great King, himself. Therefore, those Scribes and Pharisees — who are otherwise known as Lying Red Jews, who call themselves Jews, in spite of not being Israelites: because of being a Mixture of Israelites and Edomites — who will Envy the Son of the Man of Holiness for his Goodness, who will Arrange for his Death by a Cruel Crucifixion, and will Muster Up False Witnesses to do so — shall also be Born Again during the Last Days; but, behold, after 3 Nights and 3 Days, he will Arise from the Dead, even as it is Written in the *Psalms of King David,* who told about my passing through the Valley of the Shadow of Death."

05-28 [_] And Nicodemus said to him, "You must be Insane, to Think that King David was referring to you, rather than to himself, only: because there is no Mention of any Great King in that Psalm." To which Yoshua Answered, "If King David were here, Today, he would tell you that he Foresaw my Time, and how that I would be Persecuted and Tortured by my Enemies, who Naturally Assume that I am Insane; but, how many Insane People can Do Miracles, such as you have Heard about from Eye Witnesses, who have not Denied that I am in Deed that Great King; but, you do not Wholeheartedly Believe in me: because you are Blinded by your Pride and Ignorance. Yes, you are a Better Person than those other Scribes and Pharisees: because you at least Seek the Truth; but, because of your Ignorance concerning the Scriptures, you will also Stumble over my Inspired Words of Provable Truths.

05-29 [_] "Nevertheless, when the Son of a Man called Joseph shall Rise Up from the Dead, then you will Believe and Obey. Yes, you will also be one of my Humble Disciples: because I Knew you before you were Born into this World of Wonders, even before you were Conceived within the Womb of your Mother: because I am the Master Farmer, who Created you, myself, by the Power of my Heavenly Father, some of whose Truths you Reject: because you Reject the Words of his Only Chosen Son, who was Begotten by the Power of his Holy Spirit. Therefore, do yourself a Great Favor, and STUDY all of those Scriptures as if they were TRUE: because they are True, and they do Speak of me: because I have come to Fulfill the *Scriptures,* and to make all Things PLAIN and EASY to Understand." And at last Nicodemus Turned himself Away and Disappeared into the Darkness of the Night.

05-30 [_] After those Events, Yoshua and his Disciples came into the Land of Judea, where he stayed with his Disciples, while they all Fasted and Prayed, until their Minds and Bodies were somewhat Purified, even as his was Pure; but, not all: because some Disciples Needed to Do much more Fasting; and he also Baptized them with Water, after they were Purged from their Filthiness by Feasting on Fresh Sweet Fruits and Grapes. Moreover, John the Baptist was also Baptizing during that same Time, in Enon, which is near to Salim: because there was much Fresh Water there, which was Used to Immerse the People in Water, after they did their Repenting, according to the Law of Repentance, which Requires that we Fast and Pray until our Minds and Bodies are Purified: because that is the Strait and Narrow Way that Leads unto Everlasting Good Health, which few People ever Discover: because they Refuse to Believe the Inspired Words of Provable Truths, which Yoshua has Taught to us, saying: *"Except a Man should Humble himself by Means of Fasting and Praying, until he becomes like an Innocent Child with a Clean Mind and a Purified Body, he shall in no Way Enter into the Holy Kingdom of All that is Good."*

05-31 [_] Therefore, John came Preaching that same Message, in Order to Prepare the Way for the First Coming of the Master Farmer, who Arrived shortly after John, Preaching the very same Message of Repentance, which was Rejected by most of the Scribes and Pharisees: because they did not Understand the Master Plan of the Master Farmer. However, John Baptized anyone unto Repentance, even before they became Holy in Mind and Body: because it was Symbolical of that Purification, which was a Great Threat to the Evil Empire: because it Caused People to Understand what is Needful in this World of Woes, which is not all of those Vain Things of the World that one can Find for Sale in Junk Stores; but, it is Gardens and Fruit Trees that we all Desperately Need: because the Life of Man is found in the Sweet Juicy Fruits from the Trees of Life, which any Person can Discover is the Truth, if he or she simply Fasts and Prays until his or her Tongue is Clean, or until his or her Taste Buds are Working Correctly. Therefore, John Understood it: because he did much Fasting and Praying, along with his True Disciples. Furthermore, he was not yet cast into Prison at that Time: because his Appointed Hour had not yet come, according to the Master Plan of the Master Farmer, who has a Set Time for all Things, which will all be Fulfilled in Due Seasons. †‡

05-32 [_] Then there arose a certain Question between some of John's Disciples and the Jews about the Purifying of the Mind and Body. And they came to John, and said to him, "Master, behold, he who was with you beyond the River Jordan, to whom you bear Witness, has Baptized his own Disciples, who are also Baptizing all of the People who come to them. Moreover, they are Teaching all of the People that they must Repent like the Men and Wombmen of Nineveh, who Fasted for 40 Nights and 40 Days, continuously, with various Daily Washings, and Purifying their Bowels with Water, by taking Daily Enemas, after they Fasted for as long as it was Comfortable Enough to Tolerate it, according to the Teachings of that Holy Man who has come among us, who says that he has also taken such a long Fast, which gives to him the Power and Authority that he has: because he Obeyed the Holy Spirit, and was therefore Blest with Gifts. Therefore, should we Believe on him, or in you?"

05-33 [_] and John Answered, "A Man can Receive nothing from the Creator, except it is Given to him from the Throne of the Most High Ruler of this Solar System. Indeed, you yourselves bear Witness for me, that I said, 'I am not the Anointed One,' which is True; but, that 'I am Sent before him, in Order to Prepare the Way in front of him,' to which you must Agree: because I have hundreds of Self-disciplined Ones to Prove it, who also Accept the Anointed One: because we Teach the same Great Truths, and Baptize for the very same Purpose. However, he who has Control of the Hearts of the Brides is the Bridegroom, who is the Anointed One, whose Bride is the Congregation of Believers among Israelites; but, the Friend of the Bridegroom, who Stands beside him and Listens to him, Rejoices with Gladness because of the Voice of the Bridegroom: because he Loves him, who also Loves him: because he is his Best Friend. Therefore, my Joy is Fulfilled in him, who is my Best Friend. Nevertheless, he must Increase with Power and Authority: because he is the Great King; but, I must Decrease, and at last be Martyred for my Beliefs and Teachings. Therefore, he who comes from Above, from the Father of Lights, who Lives in the Highest Heaven on the Greatest Earth, is Above all People; but, he who comes from this Earth, is Earthly, and Speaks of the Earth, and of the Things of this World: because he Understands those Things; but, he who comes from Heaven is Above all Peoples, and is Worthy of our Praise and Attention. Therefore, whatever he has Seen and Heard, he Testifies to us: because he Loves us; and yet no Unclean Man Receives or Accepts his Testimony: because of his Great Pride, which will bring upon him Great Shame during the Day of Judgment, when it will be very Evident that he is not one of the Holy Ones. However, he who has Accepted his Testimony, and has Obeyed his Loving Voice, has set to his Seal that the Supreme Ruler is True, and has Kept his Promise: beCause he whom the Supreme Ruler has Sent, Speaks the Inspired Words of the Most High Ruler: because the Supreme Ruler does not Give the Holy Spirit by Measure to him; but, Fills him with his Spirit: because the Heavenly Father Loves the Perfectly Obedient Son, and has Given all Good Things into his Control, in Order to Do as he Wills it. Therefore, he who Believes on that Holy Son, and Obeys his Holy Spirit, has Everlasting Good Health, and will at Last be Given a Place within his Holy Kingdom; but, he who does not Believe his Divine Words of Inspired Truths, shall not even See what it Means to have Good Health; but, he will be Spiritually Blinded to the Truth, and will also Suffer for his Great Unbelief: because the Wrath of the Supreme Ruler abides on him, who will be Sick and Diseased for his Disobedience, even though he will be Blest for whatever Good Things that he has Said and Done.

05-34 [_] "Therefore, if we Desire that Happiness, which comes from Obeying the Master Farmer, we must Humble ourselves by Means of Fasting and Praying, even as he Humbled himself in the Wilderness for 40 Days and 40 Nights, who did not Eat Foods during that whole Time: because it was Necessary for him to set a Good Example for us to Follow; and therefore, if it were Necessary for him who was Born from Holy Parents, to Fast and Pray for 40 long Days and 40 longer Nights, then how much more Necessary is it for those People who were not Born from Holy Parents? Truly, Truly, I say to you, Except you are Physiologically and Spiritually Born Again, even as Yoshua Teaches, you cannot be Saved for any Positions within his Holy Kingdom: because those Positions are Reserved for Wise People who are Worthy of them, who are not Filthy Sinners like those Lying Red Jews, who Commit Adultery in Secret, who Lust after the Vain Things of this World, and Deprive themselves of the Love of our Heavenly Father, who Fills us Honest White Israelites with the Spirit of Love and JOY when we Learn, Believe, Love, and OBEY ALL of his Commandments."

05-35 [_] Therefore, when the Ruler, Yoshua Messiah, knew how the Pharisees had Heard that he made and Baptized more Disciples than John, and how John had Explained the Mystery of Holiness to them, he left Judea, and Departed again into Galilee: because it was not Safe to Remain in Judea: because they did not Believe in Fasting, according to the Law of Repentance: because a Man by the Name of Taberine had Fasted and Died from Suffocation and Self-intoxication: because he did not Follow **"The Proper RULES for FASTING,"** but, almost everyone Blamed Fasting for his Death: because they were Ignorant concerning such Important Subjects. Indeed, they had not been Taught the Rules for Fasting, until John the Baptist came; but, they had already had their Minds made up: because they were Persuaded that Fasting was BAD, which could even Kill a Person; and nothing could Change their Minds. Therefore, Yoshua Departed from them, and went through Samaria, which is located between Judea and Galilee. (Judea means Belonging to the Jews.)

05-36 [_] Then he came to a City of Samaria, which means Watch Station, which is called Sychar {which is pronounced SHEE-krr}, which means Strong Drink, which is near to the Parcel of Ground that Jacob gave to his Son Joseph. Now, therefore, one of Jacob's Wells was there: because he and his Servants had Dug Wells throughout that Land: because there was not Enough Rainwater to keep the Streams Running; but, it was still a Good Land at that Time: because it had Fertile Topsoil, and very Rich Grasses, which produced Healthy Cattle; but, it was Overgrazed at Times: because of Greed and Lusts, and was at last made like a Desert, when Compared with what it used to be when Jacob and his Servants arrived, whose Descendants Failed to Understand the Delicateness and Fragility of such Land, and how there are only a few Inches of Precious Topsoil, which stands between Life and Death for every Creature and Plant that Tries to Live on such Land, which should be Protected with Stone Walls, so that it does not Wash Away; and neither should it be Overgrazed with Livestocks: because that is a Sin against the Land and whomever might Inherit it.

05-37 [_] Nevertheless, Yoshua saw Jacob's Well, which was there in Sheekar, which had a short Rock Wall around it, which he sat himself on: because he was a bit Weary from the long Walk, which was about 30 Miles; and it was about the Sixth Hour of the Day when he sat down, being Noontime; but, most of his Disciples were more concerned with Eating and Drinking, in Town; and therefore, they went to get something to Drink and Eat; but this Disciple, who writes this Good News, was Intently in Love with the Good Shepherd; and therefore, I stayed with him at all Times and in all Places, and even Slept with my Head on his Chest: because he was like a Loving Father, and I was like a Loving Son, who was only a Teenager, being 18 Years Old. And then there comes a Wombman of Samaria, in order to Draw Water from the Well, who saw Yoshua sitting on the Wall; but, she did not say anything to him.

05-38 [_] However, Yoshua said to her, "Please give to me some Water to Drink." Then the Wombman of Samaria said to him, "How is it that you, Appearing to be a Jew, would Ask for a Drink from me, who am a Woman of Samaria — since the Jews do not have any Dealings with the Samaritans, who do not Accept all of the Teachings of the Jews, who have added Lies and False Doctrines to the Words of God, which he gave to Moses?"

05-39 [_] Yoshua Answered, and spoke to her Kindly, saying: "If you Knew the Gift of the Supreme Ruler, and who it is that says to you, 'Please give to me some Water to Drink,' you would have Asked for some Water from him, and he would have Given to you some Living Water." Then the Woman said to him, "Sir, you have nothing to Draw Water with, and the Well is very Deep. Therefore, from WHERE will you get that Living Water? Are you Greater than our Stepfather Jacob, who Gave to us this Well, and Drank thereof himself, along with his Children and many of their Cattle?"

05-40 [_] Yoshua Answered, "Whosoever Drinks of this Well Water shall Thirst again: because it cannot Satisfy the Spirit of Man; but, whosoever Drinks of the Living Water that I shall Give to him, shall never Thirst again: because the Water that I will Give to him will be Inside of him, like an Artesian Well of Living Water, which will Spring Up within him like a River of Joy, which will Produce Everlasting Good Health."

05-41 [_] Then the Wombman said to him, "Sir, please Give to me that Living Water, so that I never Thirst again, nor even come here to Draw any Water." And Yoshua said to her, "Go, call your Husband, and come here."

05-42 [_] And the Wombman said, "I have no Husband." To which Yoshua replied, "You have well said, 'I have no Husband': because you have had Five Husbands, and he whom you now have for a Lover is not your Husband. Therefore, concerning that Subject, you certainly Spoke the Truth."

05-43 [_] Therefore, the Wombman said to him, "I Perceive that you are a Holy Prophet. Therefore, let me Ask you some Questions, and you Answer me Truthfully. Our Fathers Worshiped the Supreme Ruler on this Mountain, which they claim is the only Right Place to Worship him; but, you Jews say that Jerusalem is the Right Place to Worship him. Therefore, WHO is telling us the Truth of it?"

05-44 [_] And Yoshua Answered, "Woman, Believe me, the Time is coming when you shall neither Think of this Mountain as the Right Place to Worship the Heavenly Father, nor at Jerusalem, neither: because the Place to Worship, itself, is not what is Most Important, since the Spirit of the Creator is everywhere, and he Hears the Prayers of those Humble People who Love and Obey his Voice and Do those Good Things that Please him. Indeed, you Worship in Vain, as all of the Heathen Peoples do: because you do not Obey his still small Voice that Speaks with your Conscience, nor do you Keep all of his Commandments, even as all True Believers would. Moreover, you do not Know whom you Worship: because you have never Know him; but, we Know him, and therefore we Know the Holy One whom we Worship: beCause Salvation is of the Judeans, who are Israelites, not Edomites. Nevertheless, the Time is coming, and has already begun, when the True Worshipers shall Worship the Father in Spirit, and According to Truths: because the Father Seek such People to Worship him, whether they are Edomites or Israelites. Indeed, the Supreme Ruler is a Great Spirit Being, even the Invisible Master Farmer and Great Architect; and they who Worship him must Worship him in Spirit and According to the Truths that he has Revealed, or else such Worship is in Vain: because he does not Hear the Prayers of those Wicked People, who do not Love nor Obey his Commandments within their Hearts and Minds, who Think Evil, who Abuse themselves, and who Do all Kinds of Wrong Things to themselves and to others."

05-45 [_] And the Wombman said to him, "I Know that the Messiah is supposed to Come: because I have Heard of him, who is called the Anointed One; and when he Comes, he will Teach to us all Good Things, and Reveal all Mysteries." And Yoshua said to her, "I who Speak to you am he."

05-46 [_] And upon the Sound of those Words, the remainder of his Disciples just Happened to come, and Marveled that he Talked with the Wombman; and yet none were so Bold as to say, "What do you Seek from her?" or "Why do you Talk with her?": because they had been Scouting around Town, Looking for some Pretty Skunks to Lust after, which was Legal in that Place. Indeed, that Town was Known for its Prostitutes, and other Things; but, those Disciples had not Found any, which they Confessed, later on, after they Realized that it was Wrong to be Looking for them: because it Bothered their Consciences. Moreover, they had done a little Drinking of some of that Strong Liquor, and were almost Drunk: because they were not Used to Drinking; but, the Spirit of Lust had Entered into them, and they could not Resist it: because they had Longing Desires for that Living Water, but did not Realize it; and also got it Confused with that so-called "Happy Water," which those Samaritans also got Confused about: because they had never even Heard of that Living Water, much less Filled their Spirits with it; and therefore, like most Deceived People, they Imagined that Happiness comes from something that is Sold in a Bottle, or Smoked in a Pipe, or perhaps Found in a Bed of Lust with some Stinking Skunk; but, I tell you the Truth, it comes from Hearing, Believing, and Obeying the Inspired Words of the Master Farmer, which will Satisfy your Soul: beCause Truths and Wisdom are very Satisfying; but, Vain and Foolish Conversations will only make you more Hungry and Thirsty than ever. Yes, he who Empties the Belly of his Mind into the Deaf Ears of a Poisonous Snake, will be Rewarded with an Intense Appetite to Feast on that Rotting Flesh with the Hogs and Dogs, and also get Drunk with those Prostituting Skunks and Porcupine Lawyers, who now Know that there are LAWS that Govern our Appetites.

05-47 [_] Therefore, when the Wombman at Jacob's Well HEARD those Words, which Sunk Deep into her Mind, she left her Waterpot at the Well, and went her own Way into the City, and said to the Men with whom she had Fornicated: "Come, See a Strange Man, who told me all of the Sinful Things that I ever did. Therefore, is he not the Anointed One?" Then those Men went Out of the City, and came to Yoshua, themselves, bringing their Doubts with them.

05-48 [_] During the Meantime, his Disciples Prayed to him, and Begged him to Eat, saying: "Master, Please EAT." Now, you can Understand WHY they Wanted him to Eat — it was in Order to Comfort themselves, who were Feeling Guilty for going to Town and Drinking too much. Indeed, they were just like all other Gluttons and Drunkards, who INSIST that you Eat and Drink with them: because it makes them Feel Guilty, if you do not; and especially if you are Fasting, and they are not: beCause that makes People of Aware of themselves. Therefore, they were Ashamed: because they Knew that their Master had not Drank any Strong Drinks, nor Eaten anything all Day. But, he said to them, "I have Foods to Eat that you Know nothing about."

05-49 [_] Therefore, those Disciples spoke to each other, in private, saying: "Has any Man brought to him anything to Eat? Does anyone Know what he is Talking about?" And Yoshua lifted up his Voice, and said to them: "My Food is Spiritual, which is to Do the Will of him who Sent me, and to Finish his Work, which is very Satisfying to my Soul. However, do you not say, 'There are yet 4 Months, and then comes the Harvest?' Behold, I say to you, Lift Up your Eyes, and LOOK on those Fields of the Devil, and See for yourselves that many Souls are Perishing: because they are Ripe and Ready to be Harvested, and Gathered into the Barn of the Master Farmer. Yes, they are just like those Fields that we passed by this very Morning, which are White like Ripe Barley; and he who Reaps those Souls will Receive Good Wages, and will Gather much Sweet Fruit for Everlasting Good Health, so that both he who Sows and he who Reaps may Rejoice Together at the Time of Harvest. And herein is that Old Saying come True — 'One Sows, and another Reaps.' Indeed, I have Sent you to Reap that Field whereon you Bestowed no Labor at all: because other Men had already Labored, and you have Entered into their Labors, and are Called to Finish the Good Work that they Began with much Faith, Hope, Trust, Love, Patience, Persistence, Endurance, Longsuffering, and with much Perspiration, Bloodshed, Martyrdom, and Sufferings of all Kinds, which you have not had to Endure. Nevertheless, all True Disciples must pass through the Furnace of Afflictions, and Pass the Tests of their Faith, in Order to Discover which ones are Worthy for Positions within the Government of the Most High Ruler, which is an Everlasting Kingdom of Righteousness in Holiness."

05-50 [_] And then those Disciples said to each other, "What is he Talking about? Does anyone Understand him? Can anyone Accept such Mystical Words, which have such Vague Meanings? What does he Mean by the Fields of the Devil? Does the Devil OWN those People who are Living in that Town over there? Surely, this Man is not Right in his Head; and yet he made Water Transform itself into Wine, and Does all Kinds of Strange Things, which none of us can Do: because we have no Power. Indeed, it must be that we have not Truly Believed his Words, nor Cleansed our Minds, which is why we are so Powerless, and without Good Understanding." And then Yoshua said to them, "You are now Beginning to See the Light, O Sons of Jacob: because the Way into Enlightenment is to Confess your Gross Ignorance, and Admit that you do NOT Know, which is the Beginning of Wisdom and Good Understanding. Therefore, DRAW

BACK those Dark Curtains of Doubt and Unbelief, which Cover your Windows of Faith, and Allow the Light of Truths to Shine into your Prison of Lies, so that you might Discover the Key of True Nolij, and thus Use it Wisely to Unlock the Door of Confession, which will Allow you to Escape! Yes, you must LEARN ALL of whatever you have Done Wrong, and then CONFESS IT: beCause THAT is the only Way that you can be Freed from the Shackles of all Kinds of Addictions, and Escape from the Prison of Sins."

05-51 [_] And then his Disciples said, "O Master, you Know that we were Sinning, just Today, when we were in Town, Lusting after some Perfumed Skunks, with whom we might Play, and were almost Overcome with Strong Drinks, until Peter said that we had better Retreat, before we Fall into some Deep Dark Bottomless Pit, from which no one can Escape without the Divine Assistance of the Master Farmer. Therefore, we left that Town, only to Discover that you had Found one of those Pretty Skunks, yourself, and was Talking with her at this very Well." And Yoshua said, "Do you not Know that if you go Looking for something, which your Heavenly Father does not Want you to have, that you will not Find it: because he Loves you; but, if he does not Care for your Soul, you can Fall Headlong into any Pit, and get Lost in the Darkness of Ignorance forever. Yes, while you were in Town, Lusting after some Pretty Skunks, I was at this Well, having a Nice Conversation with that Pretty Skunk, until all of you showed up; and then she left: because she could See that you Wanted her, and it only made her Feel that much more Guilty for her Past Sins, which I had just Reminded her of; and therefore, she had to Leave, just to Maintain her Dignity."

05-52 [_] And then James said, "O Master House Builder, you Speak the Truth — you Know that we were Lusting after some Pretty Skunks, and therefore you Inspired one of them to come to this Well at that Time, just to Teach to us that Good Lesson, and also make us Confess our Sins, and Change our Ways. Therefore, Please Forgive us, and Try to put up with our Weaknesses." And then Yoshua said to them, "O Sons of Jacob, the Master Farmer gives Sinful People certain Weaknesses, in Order to Keep them Humble and Open-minded: because he cannot Teach a PROUD and Rebellious Fool, until he is Humbled. Therefore, if you Want to be Strong, and have Power over that Devil, you must Deny yourselves of all such Lusts of the Flesh, and Keep your Minds on All that is GOOD: because it is the only Way that you can Keep yourselves from Sinning. Therefore, CROSS yourselves, and DENY yourselves of such Vain Pleasures: because they are not Satisfying to your Souls. No, it would not matter if you could go to Bed with every Pretty Skunk in this World, and Play with them all Night, every Night for YEARS — it would still be Unsatisfying: because it is Breaking a LAW of the Master Farmer, which must be Loved and Obeyed within your Hearts and Minds, which is the Law of FIDELITY, whereby you are Faithful to just One Lover. Therefore, whosoever Looks on another Person, in Order to Lust after his or her Flesh, or to have Longing Desires to Handle his or her Flesh, and to have Sex with that Person, is Committing Unlawful Sex within his or her own Mind, which will Cause his or her Body to Form BAD Acids, which will Produce Sickness, Disease, and at Last, in the End, DEATH! However, it Begins with a Spiritual Death, in your own Mind, which is Blinding to your Mind, which Prevents you from Understanding the most Simple Words: because that is HOW the Mind Works. Therefore, if you Want to have Good Understanding and True Wisdom, you must Purify your Minds, even as I Taught to you before, when you came to be Baptized; but, you Failed to get the Message: because you were not Truly Listening with your Spiritual Ears Wide Open; but, now that you have been Humiliated, you are

Listening more Intently, and you are Beginning to Learn your Lessons from the Highest School of Superior Learning."

05-53 [_] "Truly, Truly, I say to you, NO Man has Ascended up to Heaven, except for the Son of the Most High Ruler of this Solar System, who came down from his Glorious City, in Order to be Born of a Holy Mother, being Conceived by a Holy Seed from a Holy Father; but, you cannot Understand my Words, nor Realize what it Means to be Holy: because you are Unholy, and therefore you cannot Relate with the Meaning of that Great Word; but, it Means to be PURE and CLEAN in Mind, Body, and Spirit."

05-54 [_] "Therefore, I Fasted for 40 Days and 40 Nights, with Prayers for my Fellowmen, with Tears for the Lost and Dying Souls, with Mourning for the Sick and Diseased Souls, with Prayers for all of you; and after 40 Days, I got Intensely Hungry: because I had a very Great Appetite to Eat; but, I only Continued to Pray to my Heavenly Father, that he would Send his Holy Angels to Give to me the Right Foods to Eat: because there was nothing Good in that Desert to Eat; and therefore, the Angels of Heaven were Sent to me with lots of Sweet Juicy Fruits, which I freely Ate: because I was very Hungry. Indeed, I Consumed as much Fruit as I could Hold: because I had hardly Eaten any Fruit, when it Suddenly came through my Bowels, which was like being Born Again: because I Felt like a Brand New Person, being Perfectly Free from all Internal Filth, which Suddenly gave to me Unbelievable Strength, even though I was very Weak just before I Ate: because my Bowels were Poisoned by the Accumulated Filth that was within them, which had never Thoroughly been Removed from the Time that I was Born: because I had never Fasted before; but, now I was Spiritually and Physiologically Born Again, and was just as Clean in Mind and Body as any Holy Child that was ever Born. Yes, my Flesh was Fresher than the Flesh of a Child, as it reads in the Book of Jobe (chapter 33, verse 25), and I did in Deed Return to the Days of my Youth — only this Time I was Filled with the Holy Spirit, and was Blest with all Kinds of Good Gifts from our Heavenly Father, whose Holy Spirit Lives within Clean Temples. Therefore, I came to Understand how my Body was Made, and why that all People must Repent According to the Law of Repentance, so that they can also be Spiritually and Physiologically Born Again, even as I was, which was the Most Wonderful Feeling, being a thousand Times more Pleasurable than any other Thing that I had ever Done: because I was Filled with the Oil of JOY, and was Fat with Happiness, which is still Satisfying my Soul: because my Body and Mind Work Perfectly Together as One, without any Confusion of Thoughts. Indeed, my Body can now Absorb whatever Nourishment that it Needs from whatever Foods that I Eat, no matter what I Eat, if they are Natural Foods; but, the Bodies of those Fat People, who are Stuffed with all Kinds of Excess Filth, do not Work Correctly: because their Bowels cannot Absorb whatever Nourishment that they Need: because the Filth that is within their Bowels is like a Roadblock, which Prevents the Foods from being Digested and Assimilated Properly. Moreover, whatever Foods they Consume is MIXED IN with whatever other Un-eliminated Filth that is within their Bowels, which Poisons THOSE Fresh Foods, which also Poisons them each Time that they Eat, which is often so Poisonous that it makes them go to Sleep. Therefore, all such People must be very Careful HOW they Fast, and for how Long they Fast: beCause it is quite Possible for them to KILL themselves while Breaking a Fast: because Fresh Fruits can BLOAT THEM UP — like a Bloated Cow who has Eaten too much Grain, and then Drank Water — because the Fresh Fruit Juices MIX IN with all of the Accumulated Slimy Filthy and Acids within their Bowels, and it Forms GASES. Therefore, in Order to Prevent such

Gases, which can come from Eating Fruits of almost any Kind, it is Better for them to Conduct Shorter Fasts, and to Eat such Foods as Red Garden Beets, both Tops and Bottoms, being Steamed in a Kettle until Tender, when such People Break their Fasts, even though such Foods are certainly not the Perfect Foods for Mankind; but, such Foods will Work to Help Eliminate much of that Filth, and especially if those Beets are very Old and Strong-flavored, which will make the Bowels want to Reject them, along with a Bucket of Stinking Slime. Nevertheless, such Polluted People should first of all CHANGE their Diets, and Eat only Wholesome Natural Unprocessed Foods, and especially lots of Laxative Foods like Garden Vegetables, which contain lots of Roughage, which will Assist the Bowels to Eliminate much Filth, such as Accumulated Grease, Cheese, Broths, and Undigested Morbid Matter — such as the Filth that Accumulates on Unclean Tongues, and in Unclean Throats and Stomachs, which Causes Bad Breath: because the Body has not been Able to Eliminate it. However, Fasting, when Combined with a Natural Diet of mostly Sweet Juicy Fruits from the Trees of Life, will Eliminate all of that Filth and Poisons, and will make a Body Clean and Pure, even as mine, for which all Righteous People must Strive: because it is written that, 'NO UNCLEAN THING SHALL ENTER INTO THE HOLY KINGDOM OF ALL THAT IS GOOD,' as the Holy Prophet, Abinadi, has said."

05-55 [_] Now, when Yoshua said the Name of Abinadi (which is pronounced u-BIN-u-dii), us Disciples were Perplexed: because we had never Heard of that Name before; but, Yoshua said, "Truly, Truly, I say to you, that I have other Sheeps that are not of this Fold, whom you Know not: because they Live on other Lands, which you have never Seen during this Lifetime. Howbeit, their Inspired Words of Provable Truths are just as Important as my Words: because all Truths come from the same Source, which is the Master Farmer, who is the Great Creator of Heavens and Earths without Number, whose Truths are the same, both Yesterday, Today, and Forever: because the Truth cannot Change, or else it would not be the Truth. Moreover, you can Prove what I have told to you about Eating and Fasting, by simply DOING some Fasting According to **'The Proper RULES for FASTING,"** and then you will Know that I Teach the Truth to you about it, which can be Proven by those Humble People who are Honestly Seeking the Truth concerning this Most Important Subject. Yes, they can all TRY the Experiment, and Discover the Truth for themselves, and then they will Know for a Fact that it IS the Truth! However, most People are not Willing to TRY the Experiment: because they are ADDICTED to their Bad Habits, and are OVERCOME by the Lusts of their Flesh, which CRAVES Various Kinds of Filthy Things, once those Filthy Things get into their Bodies. Therefore, if you never Consume such Addictive Things, you cannot become Addicted to them. However, even if you do become Addicted to them, there is a Way to Overcome them by Self-denial. Therefore, Humble yourselves by Means of Fasting and Praying, even as King David and Joel did, and DENY yourselves of such Sensual Pleasures, and you will be Blest for it. But, WOE to those Foolish People, who Mock my Inspired Words of Provable Truths: beCause they shall be Thrust Down to HELL! Yes, they will get themselves into a Hellish Condition, from which no Man can Save them: because they are Locked Up within the Prison of Lies, being Blinded by the Darkness of Ignorance, whereby they cannot Find the KEY of the Nolij of All that is Good and Evil, whereby they might Unlock the Door of Confession. Moreover, they Cover their Windows of Faith with Dark Curtains of Doubt and Unbelief: so that the Light of Truths cannot even Shine into their Prison of Sins, where they Live in the Darkness of Ignorance, where they Wander Around and Around in a State of Confusion, whereby they Fall into Various Kinds of Pits, which have been Dug for them to Fall into by the Children of Lust and Greed. Yes, they even Dig their own Pits, and Fall into them Willfully, by their own Choosing: because they are Blinded by their Great Pride, which is Taught to them by that Public School of Ignorant Fools, and by that Universal College of almost Worthless knowledge, which only seeks to make them into Future Tax Slaves, Usury Slaves, Insurance Slaves, Sex Slaves, Drug Slaves, Childcare Slaves, and Work Slaves of an Evil Empire. But, I am come so that you can Learn the Truth, and thus be Set Free from that Prison of Lies, if you have Spiritual Ears that can Hear. Indeed, IF you are not also Blinded by PRIDE, and Hardened in your Hearts by Unbelief, you MIGHT Discover the Key of True Nolij, which Reveals all Sins, which you can Confess in the Truth, and then Escape through the Doorway of Confession from the Prison of Sins. However, if you never Learn about ALL of the SINS THAT YOU NEED TO CONFESS, how can you Confess them? Therefore, Educate yourselves with my Lovable Words of Divine Truths: because they have the Power to Set you Free from all Evil Addictions, so that you might Overcome all of your Sins, and thus STOP Sinning, as said Abinadi, the Holy Prophet, and at Last Enter into that Holy City that is coming down from the Supreme Ruler out of the Sky. Amen." {See www.Amazon.com for: **"The New MAGNIFIED Version of The Book of MOORMUN!" (The Story of the White and Dark Indians in the Americas!) By The Worldwide People's Revolution!® Book 040.**}

05-56 [_] Moreover, he spoke those Inspired Words to his Disciples, in Secret: because thy contained Great Truths that no Man Dares to Reject, lest he should become Cursed; and therefore, Yoshua did not Want to bring a Curse on all of the People, who might Reject those Divine Words because of their Ignorance concerning the Mind and Body of Mankind. Indeed, he said, "Keep those Sacred Words to yourselves, until after I have Risen from the Dead, lest those Scribes and Pharisees should Hear them, and be Converted from their Evil Ways, and thus not Fulfill their Destiny," to which we Replied, saying: "What do you Mean by their Destiny — are we all Appointed to Fulfill some Special Destiny?" — to which he Replied, saying: "Truly, Truly, I say to you, it was Appointed from the Beginning, before the Foundation of the present World Order, as you Know it, what every Man should be during this Lifetime: because some Souls were Predestined for Eternal Life, and other Souls were Predestined for Eternal Damnation; but, only IF they Rejected the Truths that have been Revealed, as most of the Scribes and Pharisees have Done, who Seek Popularity, instead of Seeking the Truth about all Important Subjects: because they are Spiritual Sons and Daughters of Satan, whom they Love more than the Master Farmer. However, you are my Chosen Disciples, and therefore, you are Predestined for Eternal Life, except for one of you, who will Betray me for a certain Price, who Loves Silver and Gold more than the Greater Riches of Truths and Wisdom. Indeed, you cannot Reject Truths: because you are Destined to be Saved for Positions within the Kingdom of the Most High Ruler; and therefore, you will Believe any Truth that I Teach to you, which is Good: because I only Teach the Truth; but, you must be Aware of the LEAVEN of the Scribes and Pharisees, which is PRIDE, which PUFFS UP and Produces Hypocrisy. Therefore, do not Allow anyone to Puff Up your Mind with Pride: because you did not make yourself, nor did you Create any Living Thing within this World; but, you were only Born into it by the Grace of the Supreme Ruler, for which you should be very Thankful: because you could have been Born within any Number of other Places that are Worse than here. Therefore, do not be Proud of nor Boastful about your Great Achievements: because you would be less than the Dust of the Ground, if it were not for the Blessings of your Creator and Supreme Ruler. Therefore, Offer to them your Praises, and Give Thanks to them every Day, for all of their Goodness and Generosity: because the Angel of Death could take you Away at an Instant, and he could Cast you Down to some

Awful Place, where you could be Tormented both Day and Night for ever and ever, just like those Scribes and Pharisees, who Reject my Inspired Words of Provable Truths, who Refuse to Humble themselves by Means of Fasting and Praying, until they are Cleansed from All that is not Right, which is Unrighteousness; and who especially Refuse to STOP THINKING EVIL, whose Minds are Filled with the Spirits of Lust and Greed, who Meditate on Ways to get more Wealth, rather than Trust the Master Farmer to Supply all of their Needs Abundantly through Obedience to my Words of Truths. In other Words, if you Love and Obey me, and Humble yourselves as I said to Do, you will have all of your Needs Well Supplied; but, if you become Proud and PUFFED UP, like those Scribes and Pharisees, then you will be Forced to Deceive, Lie, Cheat, Connive, Steal, Envy, Hate, Murder, and so on: because those are the Bitter Fruits of Rebellion and Disobedience," to which we all kept Silent: because no one could Dispute the Inspired Words of Divine Truths that came from the Mouth of our Good Shepherd.

05-57 [_] Then, when Jesus was come into Galilee, the Galileans Received him with Open Arms, having seen all of the Things that he did at Jerusalem, during the Passover Feast: because they also went unto that Feast — that is, all of the Males among them, who were Able to go, who were of the Age of 12 Years and Older. So, Yoshua came once again into Cana of Galilee, where he had Cause the Water to Transform itself into Wine. And there was a certain Nobleman there, whose Son was Sick with a High Fever at Capernaum. Therefore, when he Heard that Yoshua was come out of Judea, into Galilee, he went in Haste to him, and Begged him that he would come down to Capernaum, and Heal his Son: because he was at the Point of Death.

05-58 [_] Then Yoshua said to him, "Except you See Signs and Wonders, you will not Believe my Words of Truths." And the Nobleman said to him, "Sir, I could Care less about your Words of Truths, at this Time: because my only Son is about to Die; and therefore, I BEG you to come and Heal him: because I Know that you are a Healer."

05-59 [_] Yoshua said to him, "Go on your Way, your Son Lives; but, Understand this, O Man of Greater Faith, without Truths, there is NO Life; and without Faith, there is NO Hope; and without Love, there is no Reason to Live; but, go on your Way, and Blest according to your Faith." And the Nobleman said, "Are you Suggesting that I do not Love my own Son, for whom I came on the Run with my Horse to Talk with you?"

05-60 [_] And Yoshua said, "I Know that you Think that you Love him; but, if you Truly Loved him, you would Seek the Truths about Good Health, so that you might Teach to him how to Live without such Sicknesses: because no Wild Animals have any such Sickness as your Son has, who has Eaten too much Cheese, which has Constipated his Bowels, which has given to him a High Fever, which is the Body's Way of Eliminating it. Nevertheless, the Master Farmer has Inspired one of your Servants to give to him an Enema, which will Cause him to Recover."

05-61 [_] And the Man Believed the Words that Yoshua had Spoken to him, and thus he went on his Way to Capernaum in Peace, while Meditating on those Words that Yoshua had said to him, which he Reasoned was Great Enlightenment; but, there were others who said that it was not Right to tell him such Words: because it might have Offended him, who was a Roman; but, Yoshua said, "Do not Fret yourselves, he will be very Thankful that his Son is Healed; and therefore, you have nothing to Fear from him; but, you should Fear your own Ignorance concerning such Important Subjects: because you do not have to Suffer with such Sicknesses nor Diseases as other People Suffer with, such as you have Seen with your own Eyes in Jerusalem, where Multitudes of People are SICK and Suffering: because they are Living in the Darkness of Ignorance, and do not Understand that there are Natural Dietary Laws for PEOPLE, just the same as there are for Wild and Domesticated Animals, who would never Think of Feasting at the Table of Lust with People; but, most People Choose to IGNORE those Laws, as if it did not Matter what we Eat nor Drink; but, it does Matter: because, whosoever Disobeys those Dietary Laws is setting him or herself up for Pains and Sufferings of Various Kinds. Therefore, do yourselves a Great Favor, and let my Disciples Teach to you how to Live According to Natural Dietary Laws. Furthermore, you see how that the Nobleman got himself into a Hurry, and Missed Hearing this Message — all for the Sake of Anxiety, for being Anxious to get back to his Son, even though he Believed that he was Recovering, and had no Good Reason to be so Anxious, which Caused him to be Deprived of the Greater Things in Life, even as my Disciples will tell you: because they have also Experienced the very same Thing: because we are Given a Limited Amount of Time on this Earth, with a Choice to Do whatever we Want to with our Time. Therefore, the Wise People will spend their Spare Time, when they are not Working for a Living, Learning whatever Truths might Help them to Prosper in all Ways: because Ignorance is not Blissful; but, True Nolij is very Blissful, or, in other Words, True Nolij Fills the Soul with Bliss and Peace of Mind."

05-62 [_] So, the Nobleman went on his Way, and as he was going down to Capernaum, one of his Servants met him on the Road, and told to him what Happened, saying with Great Excitement: "Your Son Lives! Indeed, we gave to him an Enema with Water and Herbs, which we made into a Strong Tea, and then cooled it off with some Cold Water; and within Minutes he was Recovering!"

05-63 [_] Then the Nobleman went with that Servant to the House where his Son was, and Inquired what Hour of the Day it was when he began to Recover. And they said to him, "Yesterday, at the Seventh Hour the Fever left him, just after we gave to him a High Enema with Strong Tea, made of Senna Leaves." Therefore, the Father Knew that it was during the very same Hour of the Day, in which Yoshua said to him, "Your Son Lives." And therefore, the Nobleman Believed in Yoshua, and all of his Family also Believed in him; but, those Servants who had given to his Son the Enema, did not Believe: because they Accredited his Healing to the Power of the Enema with the Herbal Leaves, and would not Accept the Father's Testimony about the Master Farmer who had Inspired them to do so: because they had not Seen the Face of Yoshua, nor did they Believe that Miracles could be Done; but, this was the Second Miracle that Yoshua had Done while he was in Cana, when he came out of Judea into Galilee, which you could easily Deny was a Miracle: beCause of the Tea; but, it was an Answer to the Secret Prayer of Yoshua, who Prayed to the Master Farmer to Inspire those Servants to Do what they Did, which was a Miracle: because it was a Supernatural Thing, which would not have Happened without the Power of the Holy Spirit, which can also Inspire Generals and Kings to make the Right Decisions at just the Right Time, whereby Goodness can Overcome Evilness. Furthermore, there will be many People who will say that even these Inspired Words were Devised by the Devil, by a Man who is supposedly Possessed by Satan; but, Truly I say to you, that the Devil never did Inspire any Person to Reveal the Truth concerning any Subject, and especially concerning those Things that might put him Out of Business, which is the Business of Deceiving

People, so that he might Lead them Carefully Down to Hell, to that Awful Hellish Condition of both Body and Spirit, wherein the Body Suffers with Great Pains, Fevers, Sicknesses, Diseases, and Death, itself, in Order to bring the Spirit to Perfection for either Good or Evil Purposes. Yes, when a Person Suffers Long Enough, he or she will come to Confess the Whole Truth, whereby he or she might be Saved from all such Sins, and thus have a Change of Heart, and also a Change of Nature, which will be Imprinted on the Spirit, which will Carry that Message into the next Life, whereby such a Person will Know Instinctively what is Riit and Rong. Amen.

05-64 [_] Now, those are just some of the many Scriptures that pertain to Fasting and Praying, whereby a Person might become a Holy Person; but, only IF such a Person Follows **"The Proper RULES for FASTING!" (The Complete Instruction Manual for True Repentance!) By The Worldwide People's Revolution!® Book 046.** Therefore, do not Deprive yourself of it. Be WISE for yourself, and do not put your Trust in some Ignorant Person who is Afraid to Try the Experiment of Fasting and Praying, even if they have Religious Philosophical Arguments against Fasting, which was the one Thing that all of the Holy Prophets had in Common.

— Chapter 16 —

A List of other Interesting Literature by the same Inspired Author

16-001 "LIGHTNING Versus the Lightning Bug!" (HOW almost Everyone can become Moderately RICH, without Telling Any Lies nor Selling Any Trash!) By The Worldwide People's Revolution!® Book 001. The Cover Photo shows a Beautiful Sunrise in the Blest Land of Eternal Springtime, where the little Birds of Cheerfulness are Singing, and the Fragrant Flowers are Blooming on the Trees of Life!

16-002 [_] "What is WRong with those Professing Christians?" (A Self-Examination of the Heart of the Body of Good Government!) By The Worldwide People's Revolution!® The Cover Photo shows a Small Portion of our Retirement Home. Many Photos with Explanations can be found Inside of the Books, just as soon as I can get them Updated. Please be Patient. Meanwhile, be Wise, and get yourself some Collector's Items: beCause these are very HOT Books, which you can Discover by Reading: **"The IDEAL Place to Live!"** Book 069.

16-003 [_] "For the Love of Money!" (The Strange Things that People Say and Do to Get more Money!) The Cover Photo shows a Jewish Boy Studying the *Scriptures.* Wise People do it all of the Time; but, some go Crazy for the Love of Money!

16-004 [_] "HOW to Prepare for CLIMATE CHANGES!" (The Wisest Plan for Mankind to Follow!) The Cover Photo shows Dark Awesome Clouds.

16-005 [_] "WHY do I have to be Surrounded by CRAZY PEOPLE?" (Do almost all People Feel like they are Surrounded by CRAZY PEOPLE??) The Cover Photo shows Delicious Sweet Fragrant Ripe Mangos, which were Grown by: **"The LUSCIOUS All-Mineral Organic Method of Gardening!" (HOW to Grow DELICIOUS Satisfying Foods for Potential Kingz and Kweenz in Swanky PALACES!)** Book 021. †

16-006 [_] "The Washington Journal is a FARCE!" (C-SPAN Managers are not very WISE!) The Cover Photo shows a small Portion of Mars, up Close. This Book tells about Proper Courting, and a Chain of Command System, which also has lots of Humor for Entertainment. †

16-007 [_] "The PRAYERS of PUMPKINHEADS!" (Even God Needs a Little Humor to Cheer himself Up!) The Cover Photo shows the Author's Brother measuring a Tree.

16-008 [_] "A Sound Argument for Masters and Servants!" (WHY Everyone Needs a Good Master, and every Master Needs Good Obedient Servants!) The Cover Photo shows a Pleasant Manmade Waterfalls.

16-009 [_] "WHY are some Preachers so POOR?" (HOW almost all Preachers could Get Moderately RICH, without Preaching any Outlandish LIES!) The Cover Photo shows the Inside of a Gold-laden Church in the Blest Land of Eternal Springtime.

16-010 [_] "GOOD NEWS for REBEL WOMEN!" (HOW almost all Wives can become Moderately RICH without Leaving their Homes! Guaranteed!) The Cover Photo shows Beautiful Ceramic Work in the Blest Land of Eternal Springtime. Chapter 04 is Extremely Good.

16-011 [_] "The Low Court of Supreme Injustices is Brought to Trial!" (Our Elected King Butts Heads with the United States Supreme Court, with or without their Black Robes of Hypocrisies and Lies!) By The Worldwide People's Revolution!® The Cover Photo shows the U.S. Supreme Court Building. This Special Book contains the Famous *Declaration of Interdependence,* and the Correct Wording for the Placard on the Statue of Liberty.

16-012 [_] "The Right Design for Living!" (A List of Great Advantages for Building Beautiful Planned City States!) The Cover Photo shows the Great Pyramid at Chichen Itza, in Mexico. There are also many Photos of Swanky Mulching Rocks and other Good Things.

16-013 [_] "The Gospel According to our Elected King!" (The Good News from the Most Modern Perspective!) The Cover Photo shows a very Dirty Drunkard lying by the Street. This Book contains the NMV of Jonah's Sermon, and the Story of the Prodigal Son.

16-014 [_] "Poverty Hunger Riots Strikes Brutalities Election Deceptions and Civil Wars!" (The High Price that we Earthlings have Paid for Leaving the Good Land!) The Cover Photo shows Tombs in a Cemetery. This Inspired Book deals with a Host of Important Subjects.

16-015 [_] "Seven Great Armies of Working Soldiers!" (HOW to Provide a Way for Everyone to WORK: so as to Eliminate Poverty, Crimes, Drug Abuses, Prisons and Unnecessary Taxes!) The Cover Photo shows a Truckload of Potential Working Soldiers. This Book tells about one of my True Life Stories when I was in the Army.

16-016 [_] "The CONSTITUTION for the New RIGHTEOUS One-World GovernMINT!" (HOW all Peoples can get True Justice, and Celebrate the Great Year of JUBILEE!) The Cover Photo shows a Gathering Thunderstorm. This Book presents the 9/11/2001 Case, Grades and Bonds.

16-017 [_] "The Great World TEMPLE of PEACE!" (The Glory of Jerusalem Arises Again!) By The Worldwide People's Revolution!® The Cover Photo shows Old Jerusalem.

16-018 [_] "The Swanky Associations of Working Soldiers!" (A Fascinating Collection of Various Kinds of Voluntary Working Soldiers!) The Cover Photo shows a Malachite Pyramid. This Book is for Adults, only.

16-019 [_] "GLORIOUS Swanky Hotels Castles and Fortresses!" (Beautiful Planned City States for WISE Intelligent Well-Educated People with Common Sense and Good

Understanding!) The Cover Photo shows a Beautiful "Million-dollar" Onyx Box. This Book tells about Abraham's Tomb and the Samson Story.

16-020 [_] "Are you a Jobless Graduate of the SKQL uv FQLZ?" **(HOW to Get a GOUD EJUKAASHUN without Robbing the Bank!)** The Cover Photo shows a small and Beautiful Onyx Vase. The Book contains the NMV of *First Corinthians 13,* and Describes Living Water.

16-021 [_] "The LUSCIOUS All-Mineral Organic Method of Gardening!" **(HOW to Grow DELICIOUS Satisfying Foods for Potential Kingz and Kweenz in Swanky PALACES!)** The Cover Photo shows Beautiful Green Terraces. The Book contains many Photos with Explanations for our 100,000-gallon Cistern for Water Storage, which took 7 Years to Build.

16-022 [_] "Did God or Satan Ordain Medical Doctors??" **(Ask Huck Finn and/or Nigger Jim: because neither Tom Sawyer nor Judge Thatcher would Know!)** The Cover Photo shows Pretty Flowers at a Tomb. This Book contains the New MAGNIFIED Version (NMV) of John 3, which is very Enlightening to the Mind of Greater Faith.

16-023 [_] "The BIG White OUTHOUSE on the Not-so-Biblical Capitol DUNGHILL!" **(The Chief Sins of the Divided States of United Lies!)** The Cover Photo shows the Capitol Building in the District of Corruption, in Washington.

16-024 [_] "The Public School of IGNERUNT FQLZ!" **(HOW we have been GRAATLEE DISEEVD!)** The Cover Photo shows a Disorganized Fruit Market in a City of Confusion.

16-025 [_] "In thu Beeginingz uv Thingz!" **(Thu Kreeaashun Stooree frum thu Beegining!)** The Cover Photo shows a Yellow / Golden Sapote, which not one Person in a Million in America has ever Tasted, in spite of being one of the most Pleasant Sweetest Fruits known to Mankind, which does not Ship Well, which must be Ripened on the Tree, to be Extremely GOOD! †

16-026 [_] "God Speaks and the Whole World Listens!" **(Fire on the Mountain from the Burning Bush by the Spirit of Truth!)** The Cover Photo shows the Sign or Flag for: **"The New RIGHTEOUS One-World Government!"** This Book contains the Best Noah Stories.

16-027 [_] "Does a Good Soldier have to be a MURDERER?" **(Seven Great Swanky Armies of Voluntary Working Soldiers!)** The Cover Photo shows Danny Boy.

16-028 [_] "Thu Nq MAGNUFIID Verzhun uv Thu PROVERBZ uv KING SOLUMUN in Plaan Ingglish!" **(The Understandable Version of the Famous Proverbs of King Solomon in Plain English!)** The Cover Photo shows my Gemstones in an Onyx Jewelry Box.

16-029 [_] "UNLIMITED ENERJEE 99 Percent Pollutions Free!" **(HOW to Obtain FREE ElecTrickery, Worldwide!)** The Cover Photo shows an Onyx Tray for a large Spoon.

16-030 [_] "FREEDUM uv SPEECH!" **(U Speshoul Maguzeen uv Onist Upinyunz!)** The Cover Photo shows a Portion of one of the Author's Marble Countertops, worth 100$ per square foot, for an Example of what you could also have, if you Exercised your Faith, Hope, Trust,

Love, Patience, Persistence, and OBEDIENCE! This Book Lists the Advantages for using Swanky Mulching Rocks, and Explains Baptism by Fire and Speaking in Tongues.

16-031 [_] "A Sure Cure for GUN VIOLENCE!" (HOW TO STOP GANG WARS and CRIMINAL SHOOTINGS!) The Cover Photo shows a Short Shotgun.

16-032 [_] "AIIRMWVC and Reasonable Solutions!" (Aliens, Illegal Immigrants, Refugees, Migrant Workers and other Victims of Capitalism!) The Cover Photo shows a "Sea of People." This Book contains the NMV of Jobe 33.

16-033 [_] "Mark Twain Races for the PRESIDENCY!" (The 2020 Presidential Candidates Desperately Need Some STRONG Undefeatable COMPETITION!) The Cover Photo shows a Mountain Goat and a Silver Dollar. This Book contains my Surveys of Values, plus several Photos of Union Station and Monuments in Washington, D.C.

16-034 [_] "ECCLESIASTES UNCOVERED!" (The New MAGNIFIED Version of Ecclesiastes and the Song of Solomon in Plain English!) The Cover Photo shows a Peacock.

16-035 [_] "The Environmentalists' Paradise!" (HOW almost Everyone could be Living in a Beautiful Manmade Paradise!) The Cover Photo shows an Artist's Conception of Paradise for a single Family in the Blest Land of Perfect Oneness. The Book contains the NMV of Psalm 48 in Plain English.

16-036 [_] "The Seven Basic Spiritual Building Blocks of LIFE!" (Faith Hope Trust Love Patience Persistence and Obedience!) The Cover Photo shows Onion Domes trimmed with Gold. This Book contains the Mockingbird's Version of Hebrews 11, plus 1st Corinthians 13.

16-037 [_] "DIETS!" (A Reasonable Solution for the "Eternal Controversy"!) The Cover Photo shows some Colorful Fruits.

16-038 [_] "The Nature of CAPITALISM!" (A List of the EVILS of CAPITALISM!) This Book will contain many Photos with Explanations when it gets Updated. The Cover Photo shows a pretty Red Car. If you discover other Photos in the Book, it means that it has been Updated.

16-039 [_] "SWANGKEENOMIKS Rules the Roost!" (HOW all People can Prosper in a RIIT WAA, and STOP Polluting the Earth with Capitalist TRASH!) The Cover Photo shows a small Portion of our Retirement Home, before the 5,000+ sq. ft. Roof was Installed.

16-040 [_] "The New MAGNIFIED Version of The Book of MOORMUN!" (The Story of the White and Dark Indians in the Americas!) The Cover Photos for Volumes 1 & 2 show the Queen of England's Golden Coach, and one of our Marbleous Spanish Walls, which is Worth a thousand dollars per square yard, which is installed on 7 Walls.

16-041 [_] "The Great Worldwide TELEVISED Court HEARING!" (That Great Meeting of the Most Intelligent Minds!) The Cover Photo shows Mount Popotits covered with Snow.

16-042 [_] **"The Secret City of the Great King!" (HOW the True Church will Escape from the Great Tribulation!)** The Cover Photo shows a Colorful Ferris Wheel. P-5877. You can expect many Photos to be Inside of the Book during the Future.

16-043 [_] **"Terrorists Beware that your Days are Numbered!" (HOW to Bring those Terrorist Attacks to a Screeching HALT!)** The Cover Photo shows a Picture of George Warmonger Bush. This Book also contains the Fascinating Book of LEHI, which was Lost since the 1830's! †

16-044 [_] **"The New MAGNIFIED Version of ISAIAH in Plain English!" (The Understandable Version of the Book of Isaiah!)** The Cover Photo shows a Swanky Potato / Avocado Salad with Sweet Peas, Corn, Shredded Carrots, Celery and Black Olives. This Book will soon contain many Photos of Agate Windows.

16-045 [_] **"HOW to Become a HOLY Man!" (40 Good Reasons WHY People Should FAST and PRAY!)** The Cover Photo will show the Face of a Holy Man, just as soon as one Presents himself for the Photograph.

16-046 [_] **"The Proper RULES for FASTING!" (The Complete Instruction Manual for True Repentance!)** The Cover Photo shows an Unclean Man. There are many Photos within this Book, already, including one of me with nothing but a Fig Leaf on for Clothing.

16-047 [_] **"Are Americans the Most STUPID People who ever Lived?" (HOW Working People can PROSPER and Live in PEACE Under the Rulership of a RIGHTEOUS KING!)** The Cover Photo shows a large Portion of the Author's Marbleous Living Room Floor.

16-048 [_] **"An Amazing Collection of Wit and Wisdom!" (The Marvelous Tale of the Colorful Peacock from Angel Ridge, and the Strong Rope of Hope!)** The Cover Photo shows a Book Display.

16-049 [_] **"Justifications for Capitalizations!" (WHY our Elected King Defies the School of Fools by Capitalizing LOVE and HATE!)** The Cover Photo shows a Water Tower.

16-050 [_] **"The END of CONFUSION!" (The Great CELEBRATION of the Magnificent Wedding of the Humble Honest Nations, and the Grand Year of JUBILEE!)** The Cover Photo shows a Portion of a Colorful Parade from an Eagle's Point of View.

16-051 [_] **"The Loathsome Burdens of the Independent Jackasses!" (A New Approach for Solving our Massive Problems!)** The Cover Photo shows a Spanish Military Barracks.

16-052 [_] **"Are we Tax Slaves of a Lower Order than Lying Red JEWS?" (HOW to be Liberated from all Slavery, Worldwide!)** The Cover Photo shows a few Tax Slaves.

16-053 [_] **"The Great False Economy is now DEBUNKED!" (Adolf Hitler had a much Better Economic System!)** The Cover Photo shows a Capitalist Toilet Brush.

16-054 [_] **"The UGLY Scarred Dishonest Face of Poor Old Miserable UNCLE SAM!" (A Memorial Day Legacy!)** The Cover Photo shows a Poster of "Uncle Sam," who Symbolizes the Federal Government of **"The Divided States of United Lies!" (The so-called "United States of North America" in Disguise!)**

16-055 [_] **"The United States of the Whole World!" (A True Global Economy for the Masses of Working People!)** The Cover Photo shows a 110-year-old Well-made Mexican Rocking Chair with a Cowhide Seat — that is, IF I can get my Computer to Working again.

16-056 [_] **"The New RIGHTEOUS One-World Government!" (HOW to Establish a Righteous One-World Government without Going to WAR!)** The Cover Photo shows the Flag or Sign for that Good Government.

16-057 [_] **"Those Ridiculous Contradictions within the Holy Bible!" (HOW to Read the Bible with an Open Mind!)** The Cover Photo shows a Thorny Rose Bush.

16-058 [_] **"The Divided States of United Lies!" (The so-called "United States of North America" in Disguise!)** The Cover Photo shows a Map of the United States.

16-059 [_] **"The Complete SURVEYS of our VALUES!" (SURVEYS of Religious Spiritual Political Governmental Sexual Social Moral Economic Business Labor Habitual and Miscellaneous VALUES!)** The Cover Photo shows a large Onyx Vase in the Author's Palace.

16-060 [_] **"HOW to Get our PRIORITIES in ORDER!" (The Glories of Democracy; and, Does DEMON-ocracy have its Priorities in Order?)** The Cover Photo shows a Different View of that Onyx Vase.

16-061 [_] **"The New MAGNIFIED Version of the GOOD NEWS According to Saint LUKE!" (The Magnified Gospel of Luke in Plain English!)** The Cover Photo shows some Agate Windows. Many more Beautiful Photos can be seen within that Exceptionally Good Book.

16-062 [_] **"The New MAGNIFIED Version of the GOOD NEWS According to Saint JOHN!" (The Gospel According to Saint John Zebedee Boanerges in Plain English!)** The Cover Photo shows the Parthenon.

16-063 [_] **"The New MAGNIFIED Version of the Book of ACTS!" (The Understandable Version of the ACTS of the Apostles in Plain English!)** The Cover Photo shows a Small Portion of Arches National Park, in Utah, the Headquarters of the Latter-day Sinners!

16-064 [_] **"The New MAGNIFIED Version of the PSALMS of King David!" (The Understandable Version of the Famous Psalms in Plain English!)** The Cover Photo shows some of the Grand Canyon.

16-065 [_] **"A List of FAIR Swanky Wages!" (The Equitable Wage System!)** The Cover Photo shows a Pile of Money. This Book contains the Famous Poem, called: "HOW could we Afford it?" You will no doubt Love it.

16-066 [_] "Beautiful Swanky PALACES!" (A New Concept in Living Habits — Swanky Palaces for Poor People!) The Cover Photo shows a Bouquet of Pretty Flowers in my Kitchen.

16-067 [_] "The Swanky Sword of Divine Truths!" (The Most Powerful Weapon in the Whole Universe!) The Cover Photo shows a Lazy Robe with a Split Sword.

16-068 [_] "Has your Life become Extremely Complicated?" (HOW to Live a SIMPLE Life!) The Cover Photo shows a Retired Race Horse.

16-069 [_] "The IDEAL Place to Live!" (HOW to Discover an Ideal Place to Live!) The Cover Photo shows an Ideal Place to Live. This Book contains at least 66 Photographs with Explanations for your Enlightenment.

16-070 [_] "Our Elected King Who Speaks Out!" (It is High Time for some Sane Person to Get Control of this Insane World!) The Cover Photo shows a Part of New York City from the Top of the Empire State Building.

16-071 [_] "How GAY is GOD?" (Oh the Wonders of it all when it ALL Hangs Out!) The Cover Photo shows some Unbelievable Private Parts!

{NOTE: If you cannot Discover some of the above Books on www.Amazon.com, it just means that I have not yet gotten around to Updating them. Please be Patient, and check in again within a month or so. Thank you. Dr. Edison.}

The Enticement,

Our Elected King, is not yet a Holy Man; but, he is Working on it, whereas most People seem to be Determined to go to Hell, directly or indirectly by paying little or no Attention to their Thinking nor Eating, just as long as they are not Suffering with Severe Pains. Meanwhile, they are Missing Out on the Greater Pleasures of Living Spiritual and Rewarding Lives, whereby they might have Healthy Bodies and Happy Minds, being Free from the Torments that Inflict the Rebels and Disobedient Brats, who get their Just Rewards at their own Tables.